Environmental Health Impact Assessment of Development Projects

A Practical Guide for the WHO Eastern Mediterranean Region

Amir A Hassan   MH Birley   Eric Giroult
Raki Zghondi   MZ Ali Khan   Robert Bos

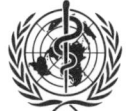

World Health Organization
Regional Office for the Eastern Mediterranean
Regional Centre for Environmental Health Activities
(CEHA)

Liverpool School of Tropical
Medicine (LSTM)

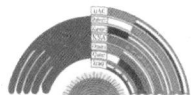

·Arab Gulf Programme for United Nations
Development Organizations (AGFUND)

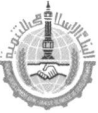

Islamic Development Bank
(IDB)

WHO Library Cataloguing in Publication Data

Hassan, Amir A.
    Environmental health impact assessment of development projects: Apractical guide for the WHO Eastern Mediterranean Region / Amir A. Hassan .
    p.
        1. Environmental health – guidelines   2. Environmental monitoring – methods
            I. Title   II. WHO Regional Office for the Eastern Mediterranean
        III. WHO Regional Centre for Environmental Health Activities   IV. Birley, M.   V. Giroult, Eric
        VI. Zghondi, Raki   VII. Khan, M. Z. Ali   VIII. Bos, Robert
        ISBN: 978-92-9021-397-0   (NLM Classification: WA 30)

© World Health Organization 2005

All rights reserved.
The designations employed and the presentation of the material in this publication do not imply the expression of any opinion whatsoever on the part of the World Health Organization concerning the legal status of any country, territory, city or area or of its authorities, or concerning the delimitation of its frontiers or boundaries. Dotted lines on maps represent approximate border lines for which there may not yet be full agreement.

The mention of specific companies or of certain manufacturers' products does not imply that they are endorsed or recommended by the World Health Organization in preference to others of a similar nature that are not mentioned. Errors and omissions excepted, the names of proprietary products are distinguished by initial capital letters.

The World Health Organization does not warrant that the information contained in this publication is complete and correct and shall not be liable for any damages incurred as a result of its use.

The named authors alone are resposible for the views expressed in this publication.

Publications of the World Health Organization can be obtained from Distribution and Sales, World Health Organization, Regional Office for the Eastern Mediterranean, PO Box 7608, Nasr City, Cairo 11371, Egypt (tel: +202 670 2535, fax: +202 670 2492; email: DSA@emro.who.int). Requests for permission to reproduce WHO EMRO publications, in part or in whole, or to translate them – whether for sale or for noncommercial distribution – should be addressed to the Regional Adviser, Health and Biomedical Information, at the above address (fax: +202 276 5400; email HBI@emro.who.int).

Cover design by Sherif Eraky

Printed in Amman, Jordan

Contents

Foreword 5
Acknowledgements 7
Introduction 9

1. Setting the stage for EHIA: creating enabling policy, and a
   legal and institutional framework 13
   Background 13
   Policy basis 14
   Institutional framework 15
   The policy basis for screening 17
   The policy basis for scoping 19
   Community and/or public participation 20
   Terms of reference 20
   Independent Review Committee 22
   The various roles of the governmental EIA and EHIA authority 23

2. EHIA policies and institutional frameworks in the Eastern Mediterranean
   Region 25
   Regional situation analysis 25
   Putting health concerns on the development agenda 30
   Barriers to the consideration of health in development 32
   Policy critique 34
   Steps towards a sustainable development framework 37
   From policy to action: strengthening existing EIA guidelines to include
   health 41

3. Observational epidemiology: information as a basis for screening 45
   Identification of health hazards 45
   Epidemiological screening of environmental determinants of health 46
   Types of projects and main environmental health impacts associated
   with them 50
   Hazards and vulnerability 57

4. Elements and methods to carry out EHIA studies 63
   Procedure 63
   Method 65

5. Appraisal of EHIA studies 83
   EHIA appraisal: purpose and functions 83
   Appraising EHIA method and procedure 84
   Appraising the conclusions 88
   Appraising the recommendations 90
References 95
Annex 1 Examples of environmental health problems from the Region 99
Annex 2 A critical review of EIA/EHIA in the Region, with particular reference
   to development activities in the private sector 119
Glossary 129

Foreword

The World Health Organization (WHO) places great emphasis on the prevention and management of adverse effects of development projects on human health, and on the promotion of healthy environments. Therefore, the development and promotion of instruments for the systematic evaluation and mitigation of health impacts of development is a primary concern. WHO's leadership role in the promotion of environmental health impact assessment (EHIA) in its Member States is exemplified by the global and regional strategies on health and environment, adopted in 1993 by the World Health Assembly and the WHO Regional Committee for the Eastern Mediterranean. At the core of both strategies lies an integrated approach to health promotion and environmental management within the context of sustainable development, and the use of EHIA as a tool in ensuring that health and environment receive adequate attention in development planning. The usefulness of EHIA lies in its capacity for comprehensive assessment of changes in environmental and social determinants of health induced by development. EHIA, therefore, provides a key-planning tool for the public sector to check, a priori, the safety of projects initiated by the private sector. It helps avoid the transfer of hidden costs to the health sector and provides a mechanism to protect vulnerable groups who, in the past, have borne the brunt of ill-health effects.

While development in various sectors in the Region has resulted in tremendous socioeconomic progress and improvements in the quality of life, the adverse impacts from these developments on the environment, social structure and health have, however, in most cases not been adequately assessed and addressed. The use of EHIA in the Region has been very limited due to insufficient expertise in this field, the non-availability of appropriate and suitable national guidelines and legislation, as well as the lack of national awareness and incentives for community participation in the EHIA process.

As part of the drive to promote EHIA as a planning and development tool, the WHO Regional Office for the Eastern Mediterranean and its Regional Centre for Environmental Health Activities (CEHA) organized six activities at the regional level: a seminar in 1991, a consultation in 1994, and four workshops in 1997, 1998, 1999 and 2002. In addition, national seminars on EHIA were held in ten countries of the Region. In 2000, CEHA participated in a World Health Organization interregional meeting on harmonization, mainstreaming and capacity-building for health impact assessment [1].

The present practical guide was developed by CEHA in collaboration with the Liverpool School of Tropical Medicine (LSTM) and the Water, Sanitation and Health Programme of WHO/Geneva. Funding support was provided by the Islamic Development Bank (IDB), Jeddah, Saudi Arabia and the Department for International Development (DFID) of the United Kingdom. The guide is intended to assist government authorities in the promotion and protection of human health and the environment early on in the drafting of development policies and the planning of programmes and projects; to provide directives on the design of terms of reference for consultants in charge of performing EHIA studies; and to propose a procedure for the review of assessment reports by national authorities as an instrument of quality control and to ensure informed decision-making on proposed economic development projects. It is also intended as a framework guide for consultants implementing EHIA studies.

Although awareness of the importance of EHIA in sustainable development is growing in the Region, there continues to be considerable room for improvement in national policies and plans of action, to ensure adequate consideration of protection and promotion of human health. It is hoped that, with the help of God, this guide will contribute to the needed improvements for a "healthy and sustainable environment" in the Region.

Hussein A. Gezairy MD FRCS
Regional Director for the Eastern Mediterranean

Acknowledgements

This guide was developed by and as a joint collaboration between the WHO Regional Centre for Environmental Health Activities (WHO/CEHA) and the Health Impact Project (HIP) of the Liverpool School of Tropical Medicine (LSTM), with funding support from the Islamic Development Bank (IDB), Jeddah, Saudi Arabia, Arab Gulf Programme for United Nations Development Organizations (AGFUND), Riyadh, Saudi Arabia, and the Department for International Development (DFID), United Kingdom.

WHO/CEHA would like to express its special thanks and appreciation to Dr A. Hassan, HIP/LSTM and Dr M. Birley, Manager, HIP/LSTM for the preparation of the first draft of the guide which was based on the available information, findings from country visits undertaken by the WHO consultants and LSTM fact-finding missions, as well as available country case-studies.

Additional text, as well as rearrangement and rewriting of some chapters of the guide was prepared by Mr E. Giroult, Consultant, Ministry of Utilities, Transportation and Housing, France.

The revised draft was discussed at a subregional workshop on environmental health impact assessment in Amman, Jordan, and was further updated by WHO/CEHA.

The final draft was edited by Dr M.Z. Ali Khan, Director, WHO/CEHA, Dr Robert Bos, Scientist, Water Sanitation and Health, Department of Protection of the Human Environment, WHO headquarters and Mr Raki Zghondi, Urban Health and Environment, WHO/CEHA.

Technical contributors

WHO/CEHA wishes to acknowledge the following reviewers for contributing to the technical review process (in alphabetical order):

Dr Hussein Abouzaid, Regional Adviser, Supportive Health and Environment, WHO Regional Office for the Eastern Mediterranean, Cairo, Egypt

Mr Hamed Ajarmeh, EIA Consultant, Former Chief of the EIA department in the Royal Scientific Society, Amman, Jordan

Dr Ahmed Al-Hazmi, Corporate Manager, SABIC Industrial Complex for Research and Development, Riyadh, Saudi Arabia

Dr Sami Al-Yakoob, Chief Consultant, National Environmental Services Co., Safat, Kuwait

Mr Sadok Atallah, Former Director, Environmental Health, WHO Regional Office for the Eastern Mediterranean, Alexandria, Egypt

Ms Maysoon Bsieso, Environmental Health Directorate, Ministry of Health, Amman, Jordan

Dr Pierre Gosselin, Professor and Head, WHO/PAHO Collaborating Centre on Environmental and Occupation, Health Impact Assessment and Surveillance, Centre Hospitalier Universitaire de Quebec, Canada

Mr Roy Kwiatkowski, Chief of Health Impact Assessment, Environmental Health Directorate, Health Canada, Ottawa, Canada

Dr Husain Sadar, Professor, College of Natural Sciences, 2240 Herzberg Laboratories, Carleton University, Ottawa, Canada

Dr J.E. Williams, Former Associate Professional Officer/Training and Research, WHO/CEHA, Amman, Jordan

Introduction

Environmental impact assessment (EIA) has been used internationally as a decision-making tool to assess and mitigate the negative environmental effects of development projects, programmes and policies. Health impact assessment (HIA) has been defined by the World Health Organization as a combination of procedures, methods and tools by which a policy, programme or project may be judged as to its potential effects on the health of a population, and the distribution of those effects within the population [2,3]. A health impact assessment can be prospective or retrospective. It can be applied to planned or completed activities of all development sectors, including activities of the health sector itself. In most countries of the WHO Eastern Mediterranean Region existing EIA frameworks will facilitate the implementation of HIA. This publication outlines methods and procedures for environmental health impact assessment (i.e. HIA done within an EIA framework), and focuses on prospective assessments of development projects.

Governments and international agencies make large investments in development. Development projects come under the responsibility of a wide range of sectors, such as energy, agriculture and industry. They may have both positive and negative impacts ranging far beyond their immediate objectives. These impacts can affect the environment, public health, social structures and the demography of local communities.

EHIA has an, often exclusive, emphasis on environmental determinants of health; it is the intention of this guide to cover these determinants comprehensively, with a focus on the biophysical factors that determine community health status. It is recognized and understood, however, that social determinants of health, such as equity, education levels, gender roles, cultural beliefs and occupational characteristics are important as well. These will, therefore, also be mentioned in the text, albeit not to the same level of comprehensiveness. Information on social determinants is relatively scarce and the framework for social impact assessment (within which the social determinants should be considered to be consistent with the EHIA approach) has not yet been firmly established in most countries. More research is needed in the Region to develop a methodology to incorporate health into social impact assessment. Another way of looking at the links between development and health is presented in Figure 1 which shows that health policies influence community health status through the delivery of health services, and development policies influence health through changes in environmental and social determinants. Also, it shows that health policies may indirectly influence development policies and environmental determinants. In most countries of the world, health policies guide decisions on the expenditure of 5% of the national budget; development policies on

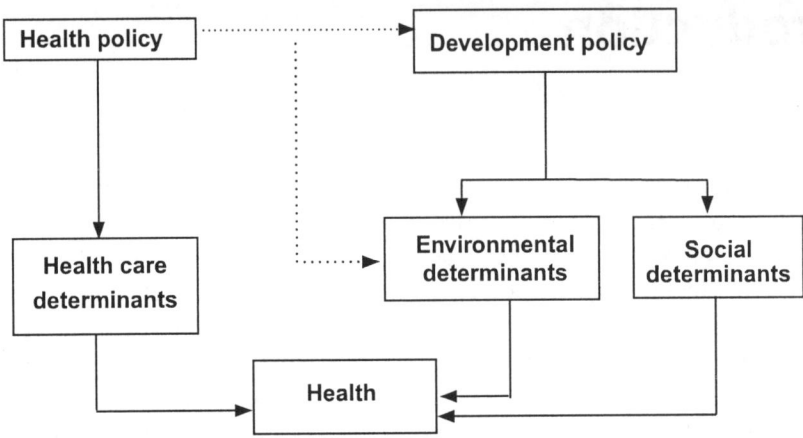

Figure 1. The impact of health policies and development policies on health status
Adapted from Birley, 2000

up to 80% of the national budget [4]. Poverty has a critical impact on both environmental and social determinants.

The sustainability of development can be ensured only if the full range of potential impacts are assessed at an early stage and action is taken in light of the outcome of the assessment.

Surprisingly, and in spite of the fact that concern for health usually underlies discussions about the environment in the development context, health itself is often not specifically considered and is seldom given a high priority in development plans [5,6,7]. As the World Commission on Environment and Development (1987) pointed out: "A development path that combines growth with reduced vulnerability is more sustainable than one that does not" [8].

Development projects, in any sector, aim to have a beneficial effect on human well-being. Sometimes, however, impacts associated with a development project may include unexpected negative effects on health. Many of these can be avoided by careful planning, including EHIA. Such adverse health impacts often touch the most vulnerable groups in society and this may amplify the overall adverse effects. They will reduce the social and economic benefits expected from the development and transfer hidden costs to the health sector. A simple trade-off between benefits and adverse effects is unacceptable; without unduly delaying development, EHIA aims at minimizing the negative impacts and, at the same time, provides a mechanism to identify health opportunities [3].

Assessing whether the nature and level of health risks may change as a result of development is the first step towards risk management. The EHIA procedure aims to identify existing and potential health hazards, to relate them to changes in environmental and social determinants of health, to interpret these changes into health risks and to suggest risk management strategies.

Often only minor actions may be required to safeguard health. The actions may vary from ensuring that the health authorities are informed of development plans, to specific requests for major changes in the development plans, such as settlement siting. At a more strategic level, EHIA may provide criteria to decide between different development options.

In summary, the health of the economy, human health and the health of the environment are mutually interdependent. Human health is seen by many as the justification for the impact assessment of development projects and for environmental protection. The EHIA procedure should be seen as a planning tool to fine-tune the selection of development options, to improve project design, and to introduce safeguards and mitigation measures when necessary. This guide aims to ensure the use of environmental health impact assessment as a planning tool to address the human health dimension in sustainable development.

The guide has three objectives:

- to introduce policy, procedural and methodological requirements for environmental health impact assessment (EHIA);
- to propose mechanisms for the incorporation of EHIA in the development planning of Member States of WHO's Eastern Mediterranean Region;
- to advise on the process of adapting the scope and format of EHIA guidelines to the specific needs of individual countries in the Region.

The preparation of this EHIA guide has drawn on international experience and has taken into account the unique regional situation, with a view to producing an appropriate tool for the countries of the Eastern Mediterranean Region. The achievement of the above objectives has been supported by a review of EHIA experiences of countries in the Region.

Outline

The guide comprises five chapters and two annexes.

Chapter 1:   Setting the stage for EHIA: creating enabling policy, and a legal and institutional framework

Chapter 2:   EHIA policies and institutional frameworks in the Eastern Mediterranean Region

Chapter 3:   Observational epidemiology: information as a basis for screening

Chapter 4:   Elements and methods to carry out EHIA studies

Chapter 5:   Appraisal of EHIA studies

References

Annex 1:   Examples of environmental health problems from the Region

Annex 2:   A critical review of EIA/EHIA in the Region, with particular reference to development activities in the private sector

Glossary

The guide takes into account the specific conditions prevailing in the Eastern Mediterranean Region, which may be summarized as follows:

- rapid population growth;
- scarce freshwater resources;
- common Islamic ethics and values;
- a state of epidemiological transition (e.g. enteric and respiratory diseases of microbial and parasitic etiology continue to be main causes of death, but cardiovascular disease, cancers and accidents are on the increase);
- mild or warm climate (facilitating the propagation of pathogens and/or vector populations, especially when water is available);
- limited industrial experience (making the working class highly vulnerable to occupational health problems);
- major importance of oil and gas industries.

This guide has been specifically developed to assist decision-makers and consultants in countries of WHO Eastern Mediterranean Region with the assessment of environmental health impacts of development projects, and the management of identified health risks. It is, however, envisaged that a wider audience, consisting of students and professionals concerned with health–environment–development linkages, will also find the guide appealing, informative and relevant.

The following institutions have sponsored the production of this guide:

- The Centre for Environmental Health Activities, World Health Organization, Regional Office for the Eastern Mediterranean (CEHA/WHO/EMRO)
- The former Health Impact Programme of the Liverpool School of Tropical Medicine (HIP/LSTM) funded by the UK Department for International Development (DfID)
- The Islamic Development Bank (IDB)
- The Arab Gulf Programme for United Nations Development Organizations (AGFUND)

Chapter 1

Setting the stage for EHIA: creating enabling policy, and a legal and institutional framework

> The chapter starts from a background that provides definitions of EIA and EHIA and clarifications of overlaps and similarities in both processes.
>
> Information is presented on the basic steps in the formulation of policies and the establishment of a legal and institutional framework for EHIA.
>
> Screening and scoping are defined and explained in detail. A checklist is provided to support the screening of projects for their need to undergo either a full scale or a simplified EHIA. The section on project scoping stresses the need for project analysis during the entire life-cycle and provides practical points to keep in mind when analysing mining and industrial projects.
>
> The chapter provides guidance on the formulation of terms of reference (TOR) for conducting an EHIA. A terms of reference example for the EHIA of the proposed construction of an electrical power plant is presented.
>
> Appraisal and quality control of EHIA procedures, the responsibilities and roles of government authorities, the composition and role of independent review committees and public participation are all addressed.
>
> Readers are reminded that these guidelines focus on environmental determinants of health and that social determinants are not fully covered.

Background

Environmental impact assessment (EIA) is a process aimed at evaluating, *exante*, the possible effects of proposed development policies, programmes and projects on the environment. It complements the economic evaluation of such proposals and allows planners and decision-makers to arrive at informed choices between different development options, and to incorporate safeguards or mitigating measures when the development goes ahead.

A recent trend is to distinguish between strategic environmental assessment (SEA) and project-oriented environmental assessment (EA). The former operates at a more upstream level where development policies are formulated and compares the impacts of different policy options. It has been adopted mainly in industrialized countries. The latter assesses the impacts of individual projects (or sometimes, in a slightly more strategic way, groups of projects, such as, the construction of many small dams in a certain area), and continues to be common in countries which rely for their development on external support from bilateral and multilateral agencies.

The process of environmental health impact assessment (EHIA) is associated and often overlapping with EIA, and its purpose is to evaluate development policies, programmes and projects for their potential impacts on the health status of human populations, and the distribution of such impacts among population/community groups. Data collection requirements of EIA and EHIA may have many features in common. Their procedures follow, by and large, the same pattern and the management measures to deal with environmental and health risks which are usually closely related. It is, therefore, imperative that they be carried out together as two coordinated activities, but each with a distinct identity and with different authorities responsible for their correct implementation.

Some countries of the Eastern Mediterranean Region have EIA procedures that need strengthening in terms of health. Other countries have not yet developed any procedures for EIA (or for Health Impact Assessment). The terminology "EHIA" adopted in this document refers to the strengthened health component within an EIA.

It is not the aim of EIA and EHIA to delay or stop projects. Rather, they aim to improve them through the design of alternatives that are environmentally friendlier and technically safer, or through the incorporation of efficient safeguards or mitigation measures. EHIA provides opportunities for public participation and is, therefore, an important public relations and information tool. EIA is now requested by most international development banks as a condition for their support of development projects. EIA and EHIA mark the starting point of a process that will yield safeguards in development planning, which may otherwise endanger the health of human populations, or the natural resources that sustain their livelihood.

Policy basis

The commitment of governments of the countries in the Eastern Mediterranean Region towards sustainable development and environmental protection comes to expression through their ratification of Agenda 21, approved at the UN Conference on Environment and Development [9]. Most governments had already shown their commitment to the health and well-being of their populations through formal adoption of the Declaration of Alma-Ata in 1978 [10] which is the basis for WHO's Health For All (HFA) strategy. Other important policy statements linking environment and health include the WHO Regional Strategy on Health and the Environment (1993), as well as two World Health Assembly Resolutions (WHA 35.17 and WHA 45.24) [11,12] which deal with health in sustainable development. EHIA has emerged as a tool to contribute to the furtherance of the goals set out by these policy intentions. In future, governments of the Region may decide to create a legal framework for EHIA fostering optimal use of this health protective and promotional tool.

EHIA legislation may address the following items:

- the institutional framework (the designation of government agencies in charge of commissioning EHIA studies, appraising assessment reports, and endorsing EHIA recommendations to the Government as a basis for informed decision-making (see the section on institutional framework, below);
- criteria to decide which kind of development projects will be subject to EHIA (see the section on screening, page 17);
- the procedure that should be followed to set the boundaries of EHIA studies (see the section on scoping, page 19);
- mechanisms to ensure public participation in the EHIA process, and regulations to define the stages of the assessment when the public should participate (see the section on community and/or public participation, page 20);
- requirements of the reporting system;
- registry and distribution of reports;
- procedures for appraising the EHIA document upon completion.

Governments may wish to go one step further through the formulation of national environment policies and/or national policies for sustainable development. This may be given shape through the creation of a local agenda 21 for local government action and through the formulation of national environmental health action plans (NEHAPs). WHO and UNDP have assisted some selected countries in the Region (e.g. Jordan and the Islamic Republic of Iran) to develop such plans.

Institutional framework

Most governments of the Eastern Mediterranean Region have established a ministry in charge of environmental affairs. Often this ministry includes a department or a unit in charge of environmental impact assessment (EIA), with responsibility for development project licensing. To ensure that the human health impact be properly assessed, it is advisable that the EIA unit expand to include at least one public health and/or environmental health expert and change its name to the Environmental and Health Impact Assessment (EHIA) unit, and that strong collaborative links be established between the Ministry of Environment and the Ministry of Health. In Tunisia, for example, the Ministry of Public Health is also in charge of the environment through its Environmental Health Directorate, thus ensuring integration of environmental and health concerns in the existing national EIA policies and procedures. This is illustrated by the fact that in

2003 the Directorate specifically strengthened the health component in existing national EIA procedures.

In most countries, the first responsibility for appraising proposals for development projects rests with the Ministry of Economic Planning. This Ministry applies economic criteria to proposed projects to assess whether they comply with the government's macroeconomic policies at the so-called pre-feasibility stage of the project cycle. If the criteria are met, it then draws up terms of reference for a detailed feasibility study that aims to reveal the project's cost–benefit ratio and internal rate of return (IRR). It is usually at this point that the second licensing mechanism takes effect in countries where EIA is an established practice, under the auspices of an environmental authority. Harmonization of the terms of reference for the two exercises and coordination between the consultant teams assigned to carry them out are crucial to ensure maximum synergies between the economic and environmental/health assessments. Moreover, such coordination will help avoid duplication and unnecessary expenditures in carrying out the assessments.

In countries where EIA has not yet been established, it will be important to ensure that environmental and health issues are taken on board in the terms of reference for the feasibility study. In this case, it will be necessary to sensitize economists to environmental and health issues, by pointing out the hidden costs incurred by adverse environmental and/or health impacts of the project.

The authority in charge of project assessment and licensing from the environmental and health perspective, generally either the Ministry of Environment, or the Ministry of Economic Planning, will be referred to in this guide as the "EIA/EHIA Commissioning Authority". It is responsible and accountable for applying EIA/EHIA policies or, where effective, implementing EIA/EHIA legislation. As a general course of procedure, it will commission EIA/EHIA studies (often in accordance with the policies of international development banks) from specialized consultants, under contractual services defined by terms of reference. As a rule, the technical and financial responsibilities for EIA/EHIA studies are borne by the project proponent. It is recommended that countries of the Eastern Mediterranean Region provide a legal basis for this rule, by anchoring these responsibilities of the proponent in their EIA/EHIA legislation. It is, however, not realistic to expect that developers of small-scale projects will have the capacity to invest in hiring EIA/EHIA consultants. For such cases, it is recommended that the law stipulates that rapid impact assessments be implemented directly by the EIA/EHIA unit of the Commissioning Authority.

Quality control is an essential element of EIA and EHIA procedures. It requires the formulation of adequate terms of reference for the consultants at the time of commissioning and a sound and independent procedure for the appraisal of the assessment report and its recommendations. To ensure transparency of the appraisal and subsequent government decisions, it is advisable that on submission of a completed report, it be reviewed, appraised and evaluated by an independent, multidisciplinary committee, composed of technical staff from the different ministries involved, complemented by reputable scientists working in relevant disciplines, and representatives from civil society. This committee should have the authority to accept or reject the report, and to request additional studies. It should also make authoritative recommendations concerning the safest project alternatives, and to appraise the proposed safeguards and mitigation measures for their economic feasibility, social acceptability and technical soundness. It will, in a substantive report, recommend a package of informed decisions for consideration by the commissioning authority, and subsequent implementation through the regular licensing procedure. The EIA/EHIA unit will act as technical secretary to this committee, whose members are, as a general rule, not remunerated for their services.

The policy basis for screening

Screening is the process by which the EIA/EHIA Commissioning Authority reviews a given development proposal and decides on the need for it to undergo an EIA and/or EHIA, and, if so, what level of assessment is required. The purpose of screening is to focus the time and resources that will be allotted to an impact assessment on the coverage of key environmental and health issues. In screening, a number of agreed criteria are applied, such as project type, size, location, and to what extent the project meets the country's essential needs.

Existing screening policies and/or legal frameworks for EIA and EHIA tend to classify projects into three categories according to their nature and size:

- those that will not be subjected to any EIA/EHIA;
- those that will be subjected to a simple and rapid assessment; and,
- those that will need a full-scale EIA and/or EHIA.

All categories of projects, including projects of the health sector itself, should undergo initial screening. The recommended level of assessment should be based on the screening results. Sometimes a small project situated in an environmentally sensitive area or close to particularly vulnerable communities can cause significant damage. Therefore, the above classification, with its focus on project size, is a guide and not a hard and fast rule. More work needs to be done to improve these criteria and countries of the Eastern Mediterranean Region will have to adapt them to the needs dictated by local conditions.

Projects for which a full-scale EIA/EHIA is suggested

- Chemical industries employing more than 50 workers and pesticide production units whatever the size of their workforce;

- Petrochemical plants and oil refineries;
- Metalwork factories with more than 50 workers;
- Construction of reservoirs with a capacity of over 50 millions cubic metres of water;
- Irrigated agricultural developments over 5000 hectares;
- Power plants;
- Industrial estates, all major industries;
- Mining industries and quarries;
- Cement factories;
- Waste incinerators, burning more than one ton per hour;
- Seawater desalinization plants;
- Any discharge of wastewater, including treated sewage recycling schemes;
- Major transportation infrastructures: harbours, airports, highways, railways, tunnels;
- Hazardous waste storage, treatment, and disposal facilities;
- Domestic solid waste landfills.

Projects for which a rapid EIA/EHIA is suggested as adequate

- Chemical industries, employing between 10 and 50 workers;
- Metalwork industries, employing between 10 and 50 workers;
- Agricultural irrigation schemes covering between 1000 and 5000 hectares;
- Incinerators burning no more than one ton of waste per day;
- Minor transportation infrastructures;
- Food processing industries and food trade establishments;
- Ceramics industries;
- Rubber industries;
- Gas-filling stations;
- Large-scale poultry or animal feedlots.

Simplified and rapid assessment procedures are usually adequate for small-scale projects, such as small industries and workshops, or small-scale water resources projects. The development of a large number of such projects in one location may, however, result in significant cumulative impacts and this justifies the commissioning of a full-scale EIA/EHIA. For example, the cumulative impact of several hundred small dams constructed in northern Ethiopia resulted in a sevenfold increase in the intensity of malaria transmission [13]. Such situations may also require a more strategic approach to safeguarding and mitigation. Usually, the main problems encountered with small-scale industries include the lack of pollution control equipment and the weakness or absence of an occupational health and safety system.

The policy basis for scoping

The purpose of scoping is to establish the boundaries for the assessment (such as spatial, temporal and administrative boundaries and financial ceilings). Scoping will help identify knowledge and data gaps, compile legal arguments relevant to the proposed project and finalize the terms of reference. The terms of reference for any EIA/EHIA should state which geographical area it will cover and for what period of time it will consider potential impacts.

The geographic scope should include all communities and ecosystems that may be impacted by the project. Issues to consider may include, for example, the flight range of mosquitoes if a malaria impact is suspected, or the transportation range of toxic chemicals, if any emission into the air, or contamination of water or soil by such chemicals is likely to arise from the project.

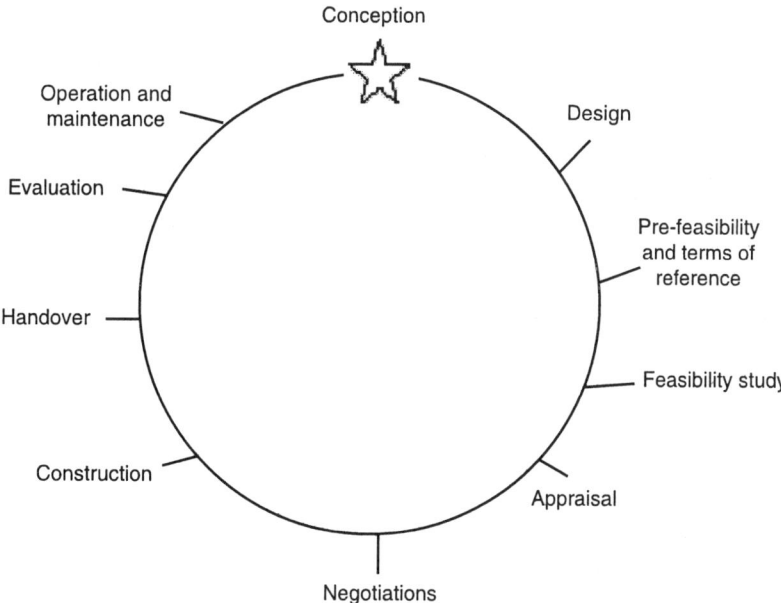

Figure 2. A graphic representation of the project cycle

Source: [14]

With respect to time boundaries, scoping should, as a starting point, consider the entire project life (i.e. planning, design, construction, operation, and, as applicable, the decommissioning phase). The project cycle concept has been described elsewhere [14], and Figure 2 presents a graphic representation with indications where EHIA decision-making and intersectoral action are critical. The output of one phase of the project cycle is the input for the next, and different authorities and sectors may be involved at the different phases. Of the decision-making points along the project cycle trajectory, two are critical for EHIA: the formulation of the feasibility study terms of reference (when terms of reference for EHIA should also be drawn up), and the appraisal (when the assessment reports are scrutinized). Opportunities for intersectoral action present themselves in practically all phases.

Community and/or public participation

Transparency should be a hallmark of development planning and basic rights of stakeholders, especially those who are affected by a project involuntarily, must be respected at all times [15]. The public should, therefore, be informed about the project with a view to avoiding controversy and to gaining public support. Importantly, EHIA legislation should establish mechanisms to ensure public participation at the relevant stages of project planning and development. Public hearings about the project should be conducted taking into account that communities and stakeholder groups may include individuals with little or no formal education. The project should be presented in a manner that all stakeholders will understand, and they should be given an opportunity to vent their concerns about the project in a way they perceive as just and fair.

Participation of representatives of stakeholder communities in the appraisal of the EHIA report is another effective confidence-building approach (see the section on the Independent Review Committee). The importance of involving local religious leaders, who have a strong bond with their communities, is also stressed.

Terms of reference

Formulation of adequate terms of reference for the EHIA consultants is an imperative. Terms of reference should, as accurately as possible, refer to the environmental and health impacts already identified by the EHIA Commissioning Authority. The terms of reference should also clearly set the boundaries for the EHIA as they have emerged from the scoping procedure. The terms of reference will not only serve as a reference framework for the consultant, but it is a key instrument in the appraisal of the EHIA report. In other words, they set the framework for the EHIA itself and for effective quality control of EHIA. Consultants must, however, be given the freedom and, indeed, be encouraged to cover any other significant impacts they may identify in the process of carrying out the EHIA, based on their professional experience. This is especially true for secondary or tertiary impacts, or other hidden impacts.

Terms of reference should indicate that the EHIA is to make use of the best available data, so as to minimize the need for data collection and analysis. The terms of reference should establish the degree of detail required and the accuracy of quantification needed, as EHIA is often based more on professional experience than on computations. A description of the desirable profile of consultant(s) to be assigned to do the assessment may be part of the terms of reference. Finally, the terms of reference should indicate the framework and the contents of the study report and a firm deadline for submission of the report.

The following list exemplifies items that may be included in the terms of reference for the EIA and EHIA of the proposed construction of a thermal-electricity generating plant:

- description of the project's purpose and objectives (e.g. electrical power production);
- description of the technical solution selected by the proponent (e.g. oil-fired thermal power plant, located along the coast, to be cooled using seawater);
- easily foreseeable environmental impacts to be expected, which have to be assessed, and other possible hidden impacts which have to be identified (e.g. air pollution under the plume of the stack, and thermal pollution of coastal water around the cooling water discharge point);
- risk assessment of potential industrial accidents (i.e. fire or explosion); this is eventually done through "Process Hazard Assessment" or PHA;
- preliminary identification of risk groups (risks may be related to age, gender, health conditions, social status or occupation) exposed to the environmental impacts generated;
- assessment of the vulnerability of the risk groups to those impacts (e.g. will workers at this power plant be provided with training, or do they have experience related to occupational risks; are there now, or will there be, people living below the plume of this plant stack; if so, how many are they; do they suffer from respiratory diseases; are there fishing communities collecting fish or sea food from the impacted coastal area; if so, what is their protein nutritional status?);
- preliminary indication of probable health impacts to be assessed (e.g. increased incidence of occupational injuries among workers, increased incidence of respiratory disease among neighbouring populations, increased protein-linked nutritional deficit among fishing communities);
- review of institutional risk factors, i.e. the capacity, capability and jurisdiction of health sector institutions to adequately deal with new or intensified health issues once the plant becomes operational;

- review of possible environmentally friendly project alternatives (e.g. is it feasible to produce the required electricity, using wind energy or solar energy?);
- review of technical mitigation measures to cope with the major environmental impacts (e.g. addition of supplementary exhaust-gas cleaning devices, design of a longer pipeline to ensure better diffusion of the warm waters discharged into the sea);
- review of mitigation measures to reduce the number of people exposed to health impacts (e.g. relocation of those living below the stack plume);
- review of mitigation measures to reduce the vulnerability of people exposed to health risks (e.g. intensive training of the workers in occupational safety and provision of protective equipment for these workers);
- review of public health mitigation measures to cope with unavoidable health risks (e.g. supply of protein nutritional complement to the children of impacted fishing community families); and,
- a proposed emergency plan to cope with the consequences of a disaster (e.g. major explosion at the plant or review of risk management measures as part of the overall environmental and health management plan).

In the preparation of capacity-building material for health impact assessment, WHO tested problem-based learning courses in a number of countries. One of the course tasks included the formulation of generic terms of reference, and examples of this are available from the course reports contained in the CD ROM accompanying the WHO training manual [33].

Independent Review Committee

Any policy framework for EHIA must include a reference to the need of establishing an Independent Review Committee, whose responsibilities and functions take effect at the appraisal phase. In order to be able to perform its role adequately, this Committee must be able to operate independently from the EHIA Commissioning Authority and from the consultants responsible for the actual EHIA. The responsibility for final decision-making remains, of course, with the Government. Committee membership will include a core of generalists, representing elected politicians, the civil service, the scientific community and civil society. Additional members will be coopted into the Commission in accordance with the type of project under assessment, and its location. These will include representatives of the communities affected by the project, representatives of business and industry, and professionals with recognized expertise on issues covered by the EHIA, such as epidemiologists, engineers and risk analysts.

It is advisable that this Committee be chaired by a highly regarded elected politician or a reputable member of the scientific community, and that the Director-General of the Ministry of Environment or Health serve as its executive secretary.

The various roles of the governmental EIA and EHIA Authority

The EIA/EHIA Authority, usually the Ministry of Environment, but sometimes the Ministry of Economic Planning, will act through its EIA/EHIA unit (or service or department); the EIA/EHIA unit must:

- register and monitor project-licensing applications;
- based on screening results, decide whether an EIA/EHIA is needed;
- based on scoping, establish geographical/temporal boundaries for the EIA/EHIA;
- ensure public participation at relevant stages of the assessment;
- implement rapid assessments of small-scale projects and check their conclusions with the Health and Environment authorities;
- issue permits of implementation for small-scale projects, with the addition of detailed health and environment mitigation measures;
- issue, or review and approve, terms of reference for consultants who are commissioned by project proponents to perform EIA/EHIA;
- provide administrative support to the appraisal of EIA/EHIA reports by the Independent Review Committee and ensure that the Committee's recommendations are taken into consideration in the process of project approval;
- prepare the Government's informed final decision for public release.

In relation to the above, the Ministry of Health also has a number of essential functions to perform under arrangements established with the Ministry of the Environment or the Ministry of Economic Planning. These functions require the creation of an appropriate policy framework. They include the following:

- assistance in the screening and scoping of proposed projects;
- assistance in the formulation, or review/approval of EHIA terms of reference;
- participation in the appraisal of the EHIA report;
- preparation of an intersectoral health management plan;
- establishment of a framework for intersectoral action (e.g. a Memorandum of Understanding);
- preparation of a solid, evidence-based position for negotiation of the health component;
- establishment of a monitoring system in compliance with the recommended measures;
- establishment of a system to monitor the health status of local communities;
- creation of a knowledge base to document experiences that will serve future assessments.

Chapter 2
EHIA policies and institutional frameworks in the Eastern Mediterranean Region

> Chapter 2 provides a summary of the situation in the Region with respect to policies and institutional frameworks for EHIA. It stresses the need for coordinated multisectoral efforts involving health, environment and other sectors in development planning and implementation, and suggests how best to meet this need. It explains why such coordination is essential for the outcome of any EHIA to lead to the desired sustainable results.
>
> Chapter 1 considered in detail the rationale for putting cross-cutting health concerns on the government policy agenda, as well as the major conducive and limiting factors related to the assessment of health impacts of development projects. The present chapter discusses policy critique/analysis as a tool to achieve realistic policies that consider prevention and control of ill-health associated with development projects as an established routine accepted by development proponents, planners, project managers and health sector professionals alike. Such policy adjustments must be seen against on-going national policy reforms related to decentralisation and modernisation of governance.
>
> The present chapter also suggests specific measures for strengthening the health component in existing EIAs. These steps, which contribute to a comprehensive sustainable development framework, can only be achieved through policy analysis and adjustment, and through enhancing intra- and intersectoral coordination and cooperation and multidisciplinary research.

Regional situation analysis

The WHO Eastern Mediterranean Region consists of a heterogeneous group of countries (see Figure 3). Geographically, the Region stretches from Morocco in the west, including most countries of north Africa, to Pakistan in the east. It covers the countries of the eastern Mediterranean in its true geographic sense, the member states of the Gulf Cooperation Council and, to the south, Sudan, Somalia and Djibouti. Thus, it covers three distinct zoogeographic regions, a broad range of socioeconomic conditions, and countries with stable governments, as well as countries with governments in transition. A binding factor among the countries of the Region is the Islamic faith and culture.

A number of countries in the Region were visited in order to document and analyse, in relation to EHIA, relevant policies and institutional arrangements, experiences and issues

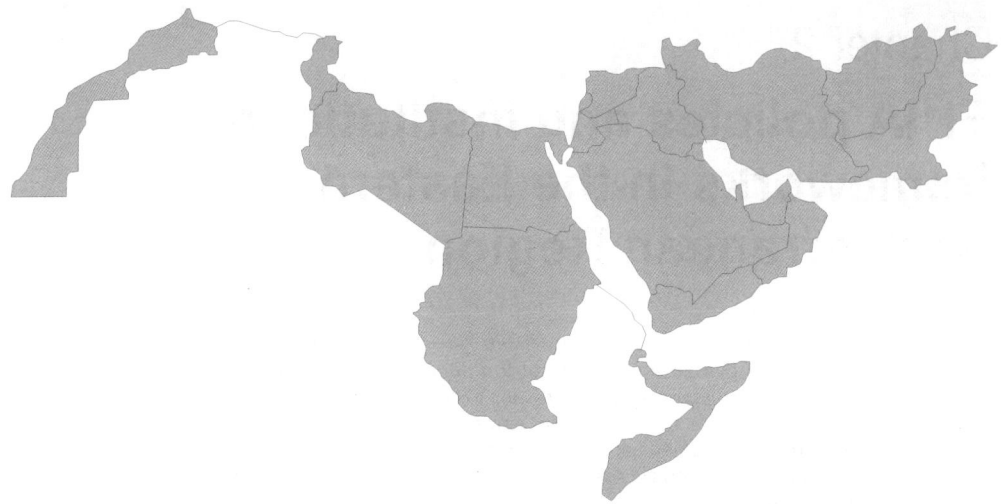

Figure 3. Countries of the WHO Eastern Mediterranean Region

related to capacity-building. Senior and middle-level decision-makers were contacted in ministries and authorities concerned with development, in the areas of economic planning, agriculture, commerce and industry, public works, environmental protection and public health. Information was collected in interviews with officials and by reviewing documents. Issues covered included:

- national and sectoral policies for the planning and implementation of development projects;
- sectoral roles and responsibilities, and mechanisms for intersectoral coordination;
- procedures for impact assessment and project approval;
- project portfolio analysis for gaps in assessments and for opportunities to incorporate health considerations;
- determination of the nature and magnitude of the main types of health impacts of development projects;
- evaluation of existing EHIA capacity and capacity-building needs, i.e. staffing, training, information and other resources required for the incorporation of health considerations into impact-related activities and project design.

As Figure 4 illustrates, appropriate tools, a sound methodology, the correct procedures and an enabling policy environment are all essential elements of EHIA. Yet, ultimately, it is the policy environment that will crucially determine the success or failure of EHIA; even with the proper tools, method and procedures in place, the decision-making criteria

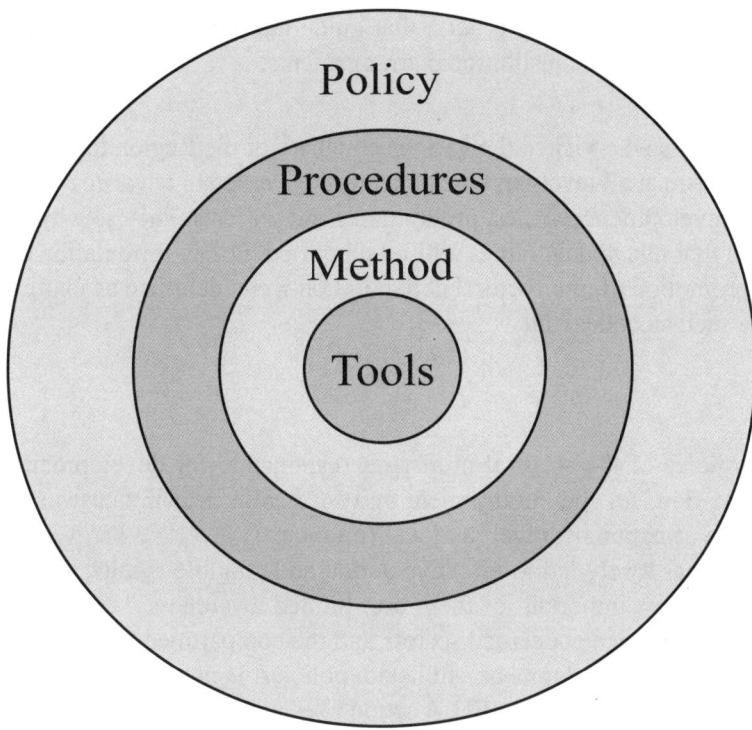

Figure 4. The key elements of EHIA and its interrelationships

applied by all relevant sectors in a common policy framework will make or break the EHIA effort. This guide will elaborate on the four elements of EHIA in the present and coming chapters, but in brief they are made up of:

Tools: environmental and occupational epidemiology, hazard and risk analysis, review of existing knowledge and evidence, mapping and georeferenced data management, application of rules of thumb and verification of lessons learned from past development experiences.

Method: screening and scoping, identification of vulnerable groups, analysis of hazards and risks in terms of community vulnerability, environmental receptivity and institutional capacity, capability and jurisdiction, risk synthesis and formulation of a health management plan, which contains design changes, mitigating measures and health promotion, with a realistic budget and a blueprint for the intersectoral arrangements.

Procedures: the management of the assessment process – determining what will be done, ensuring it gets done and applying independent quality control to what has been done.

Policy: the decision-making criteria that guide the procedures to achieving an agreed goal, linked to effective institutional arrangements.

The consultants who visited the various countries of the Region found a strong interest and enthusiasm at all levels and by all people concerned to advance the consideration of health in development policies, programmes and projects. They saw this as a promising indication that relevant activities will be supported. Policy formulation and adjustment, and the promotion of intersectoral collaboration were identified as matters of priority to facilitate such an endeavour.

Policy

Public policies of the sectoral ministries responsible for development planning and implementation, for the environment and for health in many cases allow for EHIA. This is true at national as well as local (municipal) levels. Wherever this is the case, however, it has rarely led to effective action and tangible results, due to a number of factors. The most important of these are: limited awareness, lack of capacity, lack of coordination between concerned sectors and the compartmentalization of public health concerns. Current development and health policies, legislation and goodwill may meet the minimum requirements for EHIA action. Yet, a fresh policy statement committing all relevant ministries and authorities to EHIA has the potential to give a critical incentive for such action to increase in volume and quality. Governments of the Region should aim at proposing a definitive, precise and clear EHIA policy statement backed by appropriate legislation as a near future goal. Ideally, such a policy statement should emanate from the highest political level to ensure all relevant sectors rally behind it in support.

There is a particular need to establish a strategic alliance between the environment and health sectors, founded on a solid policy basis. Within the health sector such an integrated policy framework should lead to the creation or strengthening of an environmental health department. Its mandate should reflect an appropriate balance between operational and regulatory functions and a clear-cut interface role between the Ministry of Health and other sectors. It should also ensure that intrasectoral arrangements support the flow of information and the coordination of action between the different departments within the health ministry. Among its essential functions will be all those related to the proper implementation of EHIA.

WHO and UNDP have assisted Jordan and the Islamic Republic of Iran in joint efforts of the health and the environment sectors to formulate National Environmental Health Action Plans (NEHAPs) in follow up to the recommendations of Agenda 21. Such NEHAPs also address the policy and institutional needs of EHIA.

Intersectoral collaboration

Intersectoral collaboration is a prerequisite for the successful EHIA of development projects. It is even more important for the effective follow-up action once an EHIA has been completed. There are a number of critical decision-making moments in the project cycle (see Chapter 1) when coordinated multisectoral efforts, involving the health, environment and other sectors responsible for development planning and implementation, are essential for a sustainable EHIA.

With the 1978 Alma Ata Declaration on Health for All, WHO Member States explicitly adopted the concept of intersectoral action for health. While it is, in principle, easy and popular to subscribe to the concept of intersectorality, the inherent contradictory nature of its practical application and the political realities in most countries make it one of the most elusive of all public health goals and one of the most complex to achieve. It is common for public sectors to compete over limited resources, and promoting intersectoral collaboration therefore requires deliberate policy decisions linked to adequate budget allocations that single out and give priority to actions of a truly intersectoral nature.

In almost all countries of the Region, established bodies of an intersectoral nature exist and their potential role in promoting EHIA needs to be evaluated before new intersectoral arrangements are created.

Traditionally, economic planning councils or bodies of a similar nature are charged with the coordination of development planning at the national level. They play a key role in the pre-feasibility stage of project development, when the goals of a proposed project are tested against the macroeconomic development goals established by the government. Their procedures can also identify projects that will have major economic repercussions for other public sectors, including health. Their role in EHIA can be strengthened by providing them with key health criteria that can be used in the process of considering development alternatives. They usually have the authority to reject project proposals before they reach the feasibility stage.

Environmental protection agencies are relative newcomers in most countries of the Region. They tend to be well-resourced and are often supported by international donors. There is, however, a need for legislation that gives more authority and autonomy to such agencies in their efforts to protect and promote healthy environments. In many instances, they oversee the environmental impact assessment process. Consideration of public health issues by these agencies is sometimes hampered by their programmatic emphasis on or even bias towards issues of nature conservation. Real or perceived conflicts of interest between nature conservation and public health promotion may grow out of proportion and block productive collaboration between health and environment professionals.

Science and technology councils coordinate and prioritize national research efforts, and provide a forum conducive to the promotion of multidisciplinary research. It is this type of research, often underfunded, that is so important to fill the knowledge gaps hampering the production of quality EHIAs. It is important to establish mechanisms that bring EHIA research questions to such science and technology councils for their consideration and endorsement.

EHIA is an intersectoral undertaking which cannot be reduced to an economic evaluation. Reform of environmental health departments will turn them into vehicles to strengthen intersectoral mechanisms, in situations where ad hoc intersectoral coordinating committees do not provide an adequate basis for sustained action.

No standard solution can be proposed to resolve the lack of effective intersectoral collaboration. In many countries, all sorts of intersectoral coordination committees exist but their proper functioning depends mainly on political will and commitment of the individuals involved. As a rule, they lack resources for really strategic actions. Advocacy, awareness-raising, sensitization and orientation of decision-makers at all levels are, therefore, indispensable. Whichever ministry will be coordinating EHIA policies and programmes, it will need to rely on well-resourced mechanisms for intersectoral action and on strong, multidisciplinary scientific and technical backing.

The remaining parts of this chapter provide a generic rather than a country-specific perspective of issues and aspects in policy and institutional frameworks that synthesizes the regional picture. Building on the consultants' review report, a methodic and structured layout was followed so that issues addressed can be easily grasped and translated into a country-specific context. As such, users of the guide should find the remaining sections sufficiently relevant to the situation in their own country.

Putting health concerns on the development agenda

Policies provide a consistent decision-making framework to guide courses of action adopted, for example by a government, to achieve certain objectives. They not only give direction, but they also set the boundaries within which programmes and projects are designed and implemented. Policies can be adapted or modified to meet new needs, because of new scientific findings or because of changes in the political or economic climate. It is among the duties of professionals to inform politicians and make them aware of needs for policy adjustment.

Policies designed to improve the economic conditions and living standards of communities may have unintended, yet significant effects on health. The conventional perception is that it is up to the health sector to take charge of negative health consequences that arise from policies or activities outside its own mandate. This perception has its roots in a confusion over the responsibilities for the delivery of health services (the health sector) and the responsibilities for the health status of communities (all sectors that affect health determinants by their actions). Thus, health policy is not a matter pertaining exclusively to the health sector (including the intersectoral dimensions); other sectors have the social obligation to build health considerations into their policies in a transparent way.

Numerous obstacles, however, hinder the prediction and measurement of health risks arising from development projects. Planning officials, whether from the health sector or from other sectors, are rarely adequately trained in assessing the impacts of policies, programmes and projects on health. The process of assessment is hampered by poor epidemiological baseline data, by time restrictions and by limited financial resources. The traditional epidemiological forecasting tools and methods available are often inappropriate or too far removed from the daily reality of decision-makers concerned.

It remains, nevertheless, feasible to assess quantitatively the impacts on some environmental parameters which are among key health determinants, such as drinking-water quality, air quality, food safety and mosquito vector densities, even when such data do not allow for a quantification of the resulting health outcomes in terms of mortality or morbidity.

Even when possible health consequences are considered early in development planning, this will not necessarily lead to adequate recommendations for design modifications or mitigating measures required to prevent ill-health, or to compliance with validated recommendations for health safeguards. It is especially difficult to change broad national development strategies and international economic decisions that have local negative health consequences. This is the crux of the matter because if the mitigation of ill-health impacts has to rely on health care action only, adequate resources are unlikely to be available to support the level of health services needed to control the anticipated health problems. Even with adequate resources, intersectoral cooperation in development planning is difficult to achieve. Yet, it is clear that preventive action in most cases is more efficient than after-the-fact repair.

Four major problems are contributing to the growing "health crisis" which has already increased the burden on the health sector to a level beyond what reasonably can be supported. Each of these problems has intensified during recent years, indicating the need for policy adjustments that broaden the basis of responsibility for health. These highly interrelated problems are: the expanding magnitude and diversity of the health hazards associated with development; the increasing costs of treating development-associated diseases; the depletion of tools (through drug and insecticide resistance) to control diseases; and the need for macroeconomic structural adjustment, which has resulted in major cuts in health budgets.

Forward-looking policy formulation and adjustment are required in order to confront the health hazards and risks associated with development projects; the direct cost of care and treatment of associated diseases and ill-health; and, the diminishing budgets of the health sector.

Action without prior consultation of different sectors was identified in most countries as the main factor engendering disregard and neglect of human health in the development context. A policy of integrated project development is required, with carefully planned support for health protection and promotion in and around development projects. This is especially important if health risks are due to infectious organisms. The impact of toxic chemical pollution is often limited to a cluster around the polluting source, but an outbreak of infectious disease, which is not quickly brought under control, may develop beyond any practical possibility to contain it. Examples of this include the HIV/AIDS pandemic and the outbreaks of malaria and schistosomiasis in a considerable number of impoundment and irrigation projects in the Region and elsewhere.

Barriers to the consideration of health in development

To a large extent, diseases and other forms of ill-health are avoidable outcomes of development and their introduction or exacerbation make up but one of several indicators of inadequate provision for health in development strategies. The constraints are multiple. The underlying factors, such as poverty linked to high population growth rates, and the lack of a human-development dimension in macroeconomic objectives, all militate against the promotion of health and against adequate disease prevention and control. Reference has already been made to a number of these constraints in the previous sections. They are comprehensively presented and discussed below.

- Political vision is lacking. It is assumed that paying the price of development in terms of ill-health is an unavoidable side-effect of progress, at least in the short term. Many politicians continue to feel little unease with a trade-off between the economic benefits of development projects and a certain level of adverse health impacts on vulnerable communities. The argument is still widely accepted that such economic benefits will eventually trickle down to these communities and provide a basis for improvements in their health status. This argument has, however, frequently been proven wrong. The need to sensitize politicians to the feasibility and simplicity of mitigating negative health effects should be addressed by the health sector, supported by the other sectors. The impression of "special pleading" for health should, however, be carefully avoided and arguments should be based on solid evidence and underpinned by economic analyses.
- Policy-makers in all sectors continue to be insufficiently aware of the need for and the benefits of health impact assessment and health risk management in the development context. As a result, they do not perceive the need to allocate, from the very early stages of the project cycle onwards, adequate resources for health-related activities in the development budget. Healthy populations are a critical determinant of the

sustainability of development projects. Currently, a health component appears, if at all, after construction has finished, when a project becomes operational. Policy reviews at seminars where options are discussed to adjust and improve development policies in this sense, can be instrumental in increasing the level of awareness among policy-makers.

- Wherever EIA legislation exists, it covers health inadequately. The legal framework needs updating, not only to provide a basis for the enforcement of EHIA, but also to introduce new elements of best practice, such as those formulated by the World Commission on Dams [15]. Among these feature the concepts of performance contracts and of voluntary versus involuntary risks of stakeholders, including the rights that can be derived from being exposed to risks involuntarily. Communities affected by development beyond their control should be entitled to compensation for the adverse effects they suffer, which in most instances are adverse health effects. The enforcement of existing impact assessment legislation still leaves much room for improvement.

- Mechanisms and arrangements for national coordination and integration continue to be absent or ineffective. This hampers the effective handling of health issues in development. As a first step, the promotion of intersectoral collaboration should be made a national policy, intersectoral action should be defined by clear criteria and resources should be allocated to support proposals for intersectoral action for health in the context of development.

- The health sector has not effectively played its role as custodian of health in development. The health sector is usually neither assertive nor confrontational in defining the health risks associated with projects, and fails to provide technical solutions or to identify options for intersectoral inputs for the prevention and control of diseases. It has not rallied political support that might ensure the consideration of health risks in project development. In brief, it usually does not fulfill a leadership role in intersectoral communication. The decision-makers in the health sector often consciously choose to focus capacity-building efforts on the sector's core (health services delivery), at the expense of what they consider its margins (i.e. maintaining or improving community health status).

- Health economics remains a "step-child" among public health disciplines. In spite of recent global attention to macroeconomics and health, and to promoting the burden of disease concept as a common effectiveness indicator in cost-effectiveness analyses, much needs to be done to institutionalize health economics at the heart of health sector decision-making. It is only by presenting the health impacts of development and the benefits of EHIA in solid economic terms that other sectors, especially those proposing development projects, will be made receptive to the arguments.

- In many development sectors these days the internal rate of return of projects is marginal, and the incorporation of environmental and health concerns in their economic evaluation may cause the internal rate of return to shift to negative. There is, therefore, often a well-founded resistance to mitigating measures and environmental/health safeguards, especially if they require capital investment. As a matter of policy, such measures should be considered as externalities, i.e. they should not be included in the internal rate of return calculations. Moreover, proper documentation of projects will result in further case studies revealing options of design and operational changes that can be implemented at little or no additional costs. Such information needs to be vigorously publicized.

- Donor agencies have a dissociative attitude to health matters in the context of development. As such, they pay little attention to or completely ignore health when appraising development proposals submitted for their support. This means that external support may be weak if nationals wish to acquire funds for health impact assessment and its follow-up in connection with development projects. The lack of interest of donor agencies in intersectoral issues has its roots in the strong sectoral compartmentalization of their own organizational structure. The need for policy adjustments to promote intersectoral action at national levels equally applies to bilateral and multilateral donors.
- Training and education policies continue to lack a focus on the need for professionals who can work on problems in an intersectoral team. The bias towards specialist training without adequate attention to the development of skills to engage in multidisciplinary debate and intersectoral negotiation continue to support the unsatisfactory status quo. At the local level, there are insufficient numbers of trained personnel to carry out the monitoring and surveillance functions that provide the knowledge base for proper impact assessment, and that ensure compliance with agreed recommended mitigating measures and health safeguards.
- The knowledge base for the further evolution of policies is inadequate. Policy formulation and adjustment will need to be based on solid evidence. Databases with information linking and attributing health and disease to specific elements of development projects are often incapable of providing such evidence.

Policy critique

A policy critique will support the process of arriving at relevant and pragmatic policies for EHIA. Such a critique is best started by organizing a national or local policy seminar which allows the various ministries to present updated versions of their sectoral policies and explore options to introduce or strengthen a public health component. The discussion of constraints and opportunities will help set a realistic agenda for the process of detailed policy review and adjustment that should follow such a seminar. The agenda's political endorsement, which can be achieved by inviting the various responsible ministers, will significantly enhance the success of the critique. The results of detailed interministerial policy reviews and of the development of proposals for adjustments will then be presented at a second seminar, all within a time frame of four to eight months.

The ultimate goal of such a critique is to provide arguments in favour of development policies that turn the prevention and control of diseases associated with development projects into an established routine accepted by proponents, planners, financers and managers of such projects.

The generic policy critique that follows aims to raise critical issues and set an example of the issues that may be addressed in specific cases.

Compartmentalization

Dealing with the cross-cutting problems associated with development projects has come up to sectoral barriers repeatedly and continues to find in its way the obstacles separating administrative and bureaucratic entities. Conflicts of interest, gaps in implementation and lapses in responsibility and accountability have resulted in a glaring neglect of key health issues. Yet, this has seemingly had little or no effect on the layout and execution of new projects.

Sectors exist because governments are functionally split into departments with focused missions and goals that are staffed with professionals of specialized disciplines. Sectors reflect vested societal interests, whose stakeholders have gained sufficient political influence to successfully claim their own entity in the government structure with its own resource allocation. As public resources are invariably limited, sectors are positioned as competitors and intersectoral collaboration goes against the natural flow of things. Moreover, professionals of different disciplines, such as public health specialists, engineers and economists have not been trained to share a common language, and face difficulties in communicating effectively. Sectoral compartmentalization is found at many levels, from local, municipal administrative structures (in spite of the fact that different departments often share the same premises) to regional, intergovernmental and international organizations and agencies. There is, however, a growing realization that taking refuge in narrow sectoral planning and operational compartments is unacceptable because the real world is not segregated in this way. At the lowest levels, in communities and districts, sectoral boundaries do not exist, yet even at those levels collaboration between professionals representing different sectors may be less than feasible, because decision-making about resource allocations takes place higher up in the administration.

Economic progress or health?

The narrow interests of economic development often are in conflict with those of environmental protection and/or human health. Preventive health measures can be introduced into development projects, however, without impairing their efficiency or their priority objectives for economic development. Moreover, such measures can be expected to increase productivity. Healthy communities are the key to the sustainability of development projects[1]. It is questionable whether it is valid to omit future health costs from an economic analysis of the costs and benefits of development projects.

The United Nations have developed the concept of "human development", measured through quality of life indicators, as a supplement to economic development, measured through GNP per capita. More recently, at a special session of the UN General Assembly, Heads of State adopted the Millennium Development Goals, which do not only address key public health issues (mother and child health, the reduction in infectious disease burdens), but also development issues with implied health dimensions (access to drinking-water supply and sanitation, food security and environmental integrity).

There can be no trade-offs between economic development and community health status. Any attempt in that direction runs the risk of transferring hidden costs to the health sector. The price will have to be paid in the form of increased health sector budgets. In most cases, however, no additional funds will be available, and ultimately the price is paid through a deterioration in community health.

Coordination or sectoralism?

Lack of coordination between administrative departments, such as the ministries responsible for agriculture, water supply, energy, education and health is inefficient and wasteful of national resources. Such institutional separatism usually results in schemes being implemented by relatively capital-rich bureaucracies which may, unintentionally, create ill-health. The cost of managing this is transferred, as we have noted in the previous section, to the capital-poor and under-financed health care services with their weaker infrastructure. In other words, those who create the problem do not share its real costs, whereas, in justice, those who enjoy the scheme's wider benefits should assist those suffering from it; better still, they should prevent the problems from arising in the first place.

Being capital-poor, the health sector has come to accept operating on the basis of recurrent costs and expenditures. Thus, there is a greater inclination to invest in programmes that require periodic action to keep the situation under control, rather than to make capital

---

[1] In the words of former WHO Director-General Dr Halfdan Mahler [16]: "I know that health is not everything. But, without health, everything else is nothing. Without health, development loses its most vital resource: the human being, its physical strength, its spiritual strength".

investments in infrastructure that will eliminate health risks once and for all. This has also led to a disproportionate bias towards operational action at the expense of a regulatory role whereby the health sector can force other sectors to ensure their actions are least harmful to health. This bias comes to expression in the relative weakness of environmental and occupational health departments.

Failure to implement international agreements on health protection

There is no lack of memoranda of understanding and agreements on collaboration between international organizations. These agreements take a short-term view and usually lack the executive and administrative support necessary for implementation. Nevertheless, they provide a basis for action and their strengthening should be a matter of priority for Member States and be emulated by them at the national level between authorities that would benefit from the coordination of efforts.

Similarly, there are no lack of guidelines, yet they are seldom put to use, and never to their full potential. A shift in focus from the continued process of updating and expanding guidelines could be achieved by a policy that ensures well-evidenced and time-proven guidelines are actually made to be an integral part of contracts for development projects. Not applying the rules of good practice they provide should imply a breach of contract that can be countered by proper sanctions.

Steps towards a sustainable development framework

The steps outlined below will lead to a framework for EHIA policy decisions and, through them, to programmes and action. Policy adjustment is required to confront the health hazards and risks associated with development projects, to take account of the direct cost of care and treatment of development-associated ill-health and the diminishing budgets of the health sector. The steps described address different approaches to achieving policy adjustment.

First principle

The principle has to be established that economic development should not create ill-health or contribute to inequity in health status between different communities. Development projects should allow for health protection and promotion at all stages of planning, design, building, operation and decommissioning, with special reference to vulnerable groups.

Impact assessment

As a matter of policy, each proposed scheme should be preceded by a screening and scoping exercise, followed by an analysis and evaluation of the findings in terms of potential impacts on health as well as their economic dimensions. The assessment has to be holistic and multidisciplinary. It should identify unintended negative side-effects on health that could be anticipated and provide economic evaluation of prevention, treatment and control measures. It should also identify the opportunities for health promotion that can be effectively seized in the context of the project. Experience and outcome should feed into the process of a rolling revision of EHIA guidelines.

Monitoring, evaluation, and response

A critical policy area relates to the generation of capacity to respond to problems as they arise. A continuing programme that monitors ecosystems, health determinants and human health status, with specific lines of reporting and administrative mechanisms for action, should be incorporated into each development project. The investigations would be on a small scale and modestly funded. In large institutionalized schemes, a multidisciplinary unit could be established to investigate and improve disease prevention and control. Another, related policy area is that of monitoring compliance with recommended health safeguards, mitigating measures and health promotional activities.

Creation of national authorities

The fundamental requirements for intersectoral collaboration make it imperative to place responsibility for EHIA at the highest possible administrative level. National EHIA authorities should have executive power, backed up directly by the cabinet, the Prime Minister's Office or the President's Office, so as to promote cooperation between ministries responsible for public works, energy, industry, agriculture, education, health and transport, and other related bodies. Intersectoral cooperation would be a matter of best practice, and could be further enhanced by the earmarking of government funds exclusively for intersectoral action. Strict criteria would have to apply for the allocation of such resources.

Integrated development strategies

Multisectoral planning. Only through integrated multisectoral planning is it possible to achieve all the goals of development including improved health. The World Bank and the regional development banks support the principle of "do no harm" and subscribe to the concept that ill-health impacts can be quantified by the loss of DALYs (disability-adjusted life years) for the sake of costing and integration into cost–benefit analysis.

The endorsement of these concepts by multilateral finance agencies is gradually finding resonance in the commercial banking world as well, and through these in corporate industry.

Guidelines. Guidelines on integrated development planning, eventually leading to specific technical manuals, should cover health planning. The health component in such guidelines should be concise, explicit and widely applicable, and should include recommendations for the creation of multidisciplinary planning teams.

Coordination. It is necessary to integrate sectoral planning for agronomy, ecology, economics, environmental monitoring, epidemiology, health services, health surveillance, housing, hygiene, hydrology, social activity, pest and vector management, wildlife ecology and unplanned or "spontaneous" settlements. Just as intersectoral coordination is required in integrated development planning, regional or spatial coordination is equally necessary as impacts from development projects do not respect political boundaries, the so-called transboundary effects.

National standards

National regulations. Development schemes should conform to national guidelines or regulations where these exist. Countries should develop regulations for the continuous evaluation of health impacts. In other words, the regulations should cover health impact evaluation during the entire project life (life-cycle assessment).

National registration. There is a growing awareness of the need to better understand both current and projected growth rates in the construction of large and small development schemes. A lack of information and documentation of these developments becomes increasingly disquieting to health officials confronted by the disease effects. National registers of projects and their health impacts would be useful in this respect and would support the early recognition of specific problems. Past experience in comparable settings is the single most solid input into an EHIA.

Financial support

Conditional financing. Applications for grants and loans for development projects should be carefully scrutinized by national authorities and donor agencies to ensure that they conform to national regulations for health promotion and to international regulations when national regulations are not sufficient. They should also be screened for their opportunities to further extend EHIA capacity-building.

Costs of the health care infrastructure. Capital costs of the necessary health care infrastructure, such as for buildings, clinics, outpatient facilities and so on, should not be included in the integrated capital costs of projects. The aforementioned negative impact on the internal rate of return provides a strong argument to consider them as externalities. Greater transparency is another powerful argument; situations should be avoided where essential project components (such as drainage works for an irrigation scheme) are labelled as health components. The costs of recruiting and training teams of health care professionals for rural areas should be included from the outset. Additional health care personnel are not, as a rule, immediately available to meet the extra demands created by new projects, and a training scheme is normally needed.

Recurrent costs for health services, screening, treatment, control and health education should be covered in standard budget planning. The funds required for recurrent operational expenditure should be derived directly or indirectly from gross income. This should be done on an as-needed basis or on some equivalency basis, for instance, by taking a fixed proportion of project income. Recurrent costs should also include those of regular health surveillance and evaluation and of environmental monitoring.

Conclusions of the policy critique

There is a widespread awareness in the Region of the dangers of environmental degradation, but this does not guarantee that the associated health issues will be adequately mitigated. Development cannot be expected automatically to confine its harmful impact on health to socially, economically or even politically acceptable levels. In the context of development, the level of concern devoted by policy-makers to environmental issues seems disproportionate in comparison with the level of concern devoted to human health.

A health budget adjustment or even increase favouring regulatory functions would allow part of the development budgets to be tapped for health protection and promotion.

The health sector should prepare operational plans for the utilization of external resources available to projects, in order to improve general health services and to achieve disease prevention and control. The responsibilities of all parties concerned should be agreed so as to ensure coordinated implementation.

The available tools, although not complete, are sufficient to justify action. Action is needed to reform and adjust policy, institutional arrangements, the planning process for development projects, and the environmental impact assessment (EIA) guidelines and associated procedures so as to ensure that human health is fully taken into account.

From policy to action: strengthening existing EIA guidelines to include health

Changing the definition of EIA

To many EIA practitioners, the ultimate reason for assessing environmental impacts is to safeguard the health of people. Yet many current definitions of EIA fail to refer to human health in an appropriate way. The most likely reason for this is that those designing EIA's have a sectoral concept of health, which is unfortunately often reinforced by the core of the health sector itself. Poisoning and noncommunicable diseases associated with chemicals in air, water and soil, and organic pollution of drinking-water top the list of EIA health issues. This bias reflects the industrialized country origins of EIA. There are, however, many other health concerns, including: malnutrition, injury and psychosocial disorder, as well as the more traditional communicable diseases. In specific settings, certainly also in the EMR countries, these other health concerns are often equally or more important and acute than the health effects of residual pollution.

EIA is undertaken in response to environmental laws that have been enacted in many countries. These often contain a definition of the environment that is too narrow. The definition should include human communities and their health. A typical definition is "the sphere in which man and other creatures live". This could be changed to "the sphere in which people and other creatures live and have their well-being, and on which they depend for their livelihood and sustainable survival". EIA/EHIA is usually part of the planning process of new projects. It may, however, also be important to assess the environmental and health impacts of existing projects and document the results in a national EHIA knowledge base.

The first step in strengthening EIA guidelines is simply to include an explicit reference to human health. This reference can be repeated at each step of the assessment procedure. For example:

- consider health aspects during the process of screening;
- during the scoping step, make reference to environmental and health concerns;
- include health, economy and well-being in the analysis of stakeholder effects;
- collect data required to identify and assess the main effects that the project is likely to have on the environment and human health;
- require EIA reports to summarize health statistics and comment on their limitations;

- require environmental management plans to comment on the capability of environmental units and health units at the site of the project;
- include the requirement for a separate, intersectoral health management plan;
- require monitoring plans to refer to health indicators or proxy health indicators and include occupational health and safety;
- include public health or environmental health officers in EHIA appraisal procedures as a matter of standard practice.

Many guidelines list the types of impacts that are of interest, often referring to World Bank Sourcebooks. Unfortunately, the original editions of these sourcebooks did not cover health impacts among a range of other issues. Through the publication of a series of updates the Bank has now rectified this. One of these incorporates human health [17][2]. The reader will also find in Chapter 4 of this guide, examples of the most significant health impacts to be expected from the most common projects developed in the Region.

Identification of impacts

EIA regulations usually contain a procedure for screening projects and assigning them to one of two or more categories (e.g. Tunisia, Egypt). In the case of two categories, usually the first one lists projects that are sufficiently sensitive to require a full-scale EIA. The second category lists projects that may require a simplified EIA. These lists should be revised to consider whether the project could have a significant impact on people's health and well-being. For example, using these criteria, projects designed for the use of wastewater in agriculture should be upgraded to the list of projects that should be subject to a full-scale EIA. Examples of lists appropriate to the Region can be found in Chapter 1.

Responsibilities of EIA units

EIA units are usually situated in environment ministries or environmental protection agencies rather than in health ministries. This makes sense and is appropriate. There has been a natural evolution of the responsibilities of environmental health officers in many countries. Such officers are often stationed in departments other than health, where they can provide a specialist monitoring role. The officers recruited to EIA units may

---

[2] The HIA update can be found on http://lnweb18.worldbank.org/essd/essd.nsf/0/88ea207ffa800d27852567f5005b37ae/$FILE/ATTHSQ3N/eano18.pdf

frequently come from an environmental health background. In any event, the general responsibilities of an EIA unit should include:

- reviewing and studying environmental problems and health problems with predominantly environmental determinants;
- assessing hazards and risks linked to the release of chemicals or radiation;
- controlling all activities with actual or potential impacts on the environment and human health.

Its specific responsibilities will be:

- to decide whether a specific project will need a full-scale EHIA, or only a rapid assessment of its health impact, or nothing at all. This function should be anchored in the EIA/EHIA legislation;
- to draft relevant and accurate terms of reference for consultants entrusted to perform EHIA studies;
- to appraise EHIA reports prepared by consultants;
- eventually to perform rapid assessments as referred to in Chapter 1.

The EIA unit needs to be staffed with experts specialized in relevant disciplines; often this will include a social scientist, a water quality expert, an air quality expert, a soil scientist, an ecologist and a public health specialist.

Similarly, officers responsible for monitoring environmental quality are not confined to EIA units but may also be found in environmental health units at the Ministry of Health, and in occupational health and safety units at the Ministry of Labour. Different levels of decentralization in different sectors may hamper communications between these professionals, but once effective communication channels have been established, their presence at different levels may add a valuable dimension to their mutual complementarity.

Standards

Standards exist for the maximum discharge and intake of many pollutants and these form an important basis for EIA. The standards are derived from toxicological or other biomedical research. Unfortunately, for many project components that have a health impact no such standards exist. There are also cases where standards exist but are not included in EIA, such as occupational health and safety.

Basically, if pollution levels resulting from any project are compatible with broadly accepted standards (such as the limit values included in WHO guidelines for air or drinking-water quality), then it will be considered that this project has no significant health impact through those important pathways of exposure (air and drinking-water).

Terms of reference

One of the most crucial preconditions for including more explicit concerns for human health in the EIA procedure is the strengthening of the health component in existing EIA terms of reference. The terms of reference are provided to the consultants who conduct the EIA by the project proponents under the supervision of the regulatory agency, or directly by this regulatory agency. The terms of reference should include specific references to human health with subheadings to address at least the following points:

- hazard identification;
- vulnerable communities;
- community risk factors;
- environmental factors;
- institutional risk factors;
- health risk management;
- cumulative effects.

Regarding cumulative effects, it is now widely recognized that while individual industries, for example, may produce low levels of pollutants, exposure can be cumulative with time. Pollution levels may also be spatially cumulative when numerous small-scale industries are located in the same place. This can only be handled satisfactorily by an EIA that considers the entire air- or watershed. For this reason, strategic impact assessments are becoming more popular and health concerns need to be explicitly articulated.

Chapter 3
Observational epidemiology: information as a basis for screening

> This chapter is intended to remind readers, in particular members of national EIA/EHIA commissioning authorities, of the range of health hazards and the variety of development projects they need to consider. It has been written to assist scientists with different disciplinary backgrounds, especially environmental engineers and public health specialists, to gain an improved understanding of each other's fields. It focuses on project screening. The information provided draws on illustrative examples from the Region.
>
> In principle, screening of development proposals is a desk exercise, guided by a number of criteria, available data and the expertise present in a generalist team. Only in exceptional cases will it include a field visit. National EIA/EHIA commissioning authorities will need to have the capacity to screen a relatively high volume of proposals over relatively short periods of time, based on agreed criteria, and to formulate terms of reference for those cases that are deemed to require a full EHIA.
>
> Adequate decision-making at the end of the screening process demands that for each project all possible health hazards are considered. A comprehensive overview of hazards is presented below, in association with their critical environmental determinants. The process of hazard identification is further facilitated by a listing of different types of projects, and the health hazards that are associated with them. Finally, some of the most obvious changes in environmental determinants of health are considered in relation to vulnerable groups.

Identification of health hazards

Three categories of significant health hazards may be distinguished:

- the concentration of toxic or carcinogenic physical and/or chemical pollutants in air, water or soil;
- the presence of microbiological pathogens, and/or enhancement of one or more pathways of human infection open to these pathogenic organisms;
- loss of major life-sustaining resources, such as fresh water, productive lands or fisheries;

Within the Eastern Mediterranean Region:

- Excessive concentrations of toxic chemicals will be found mostly in the vicinity of industrial and mining projects, but they may also occur in relation to cottage industries and in consumer goods.
- Infectious diseases are a major public health issue and infectious organisms are responsible for important disease burdens.

- Population movement facilitates the spread of pathogenic organisms.
- Any increase of uncontrolled wet areas will enhance the propagation of waterborne pathogens and of water-associated vectors of viruses and parasites.
- Uncontrolled discharges of raw sewage or of human excreta will carry the risk of an increase in the transmission of enteric infections through water or food.
- The main endangered life-sustaining resources will be underground and surface freshwater resources, but the loss of good agricultural lands or of fisheries may also have major detrimental impacts on the nutritional status of human populations.

Epidemiological screening of environmental determinants of health

The following section is intended especially for engineers and infrastructure specialists contributing to EHIA screening. It provides a brief introduction to a number of health hazards.

Endemic parasitic disease hazards

In the Eastern Mediterranean Region, the four parasitic diseases malaria, schistosomiasis, leishmaniasis and lymphatic filariasis are significantly prevalent. These diseases are responsible for significant health burdens in several areas. The critical environmental determinants are illustrated by the following examples.

- The malaria parasite is a main endemic parasitic hazard in most countries, with mosquitoes of the genus *Anopheles* as its vector. Any water impoundment (pond, reservoir or man-made lake) that leads to an increase in the anopheline mosquito population density, or creates conditions contributing to an increased longevity of vectors, may therefore increase the risk of malaria transmission to local populations exposed to mosquito bites.
- Schistosomiasis is especially prevalent all along the Nile river, but also has a history of foci in Morocco and the Islamic Republic of Iran, among other countries. Expansion of irrigated agriculture in infested areas may increase suitable habitats for the aquatic snail species that are the intermediate hosts of the larvae of *Schistosoma* parasites. Such environmental changes therefore increase the risk of schistosomiasis transmission to farming populations working in contact with waters where the infectious larvae of the parasite (cercariae) occur.
- Any change in rangelands that enhances the growth of shrubs on which rural rodents feed, may lead to an expansion of the populations of intermediate hosts of the *Leishmania* parasite and therefore to an increased risk of leishmaniasis transmission to the human population living in their proximity.

- *Culex* mosquitoes, vectors of lymphatic filariasis, breed by preference in organically polluted waters. The creation of stabilization ponds, ditches with stagnant sewage and other collections of organically polluted water will indirectly increase the risk of local filariasis transmission.

In the Eastern Mediterranean Region, malaria-infected areas and schistosomiasis-infected areas are recorded on WHO epidemiological maps, and are well known by national health authorities. These authorities are also well informed about the range of leishmaniasis-infected areas. Filariasis, however, is only a marginal problem in the Region, limited to southern Sudan, Djibouti and Somalia. Filariasis may nevertheless gain in significance as there is a risk of its importation from southern Asia to Gulf Cooperation Council countries through migrant workers, whenever the existing health screening system applied in the recruitment of those workers underperforms. In addition, more favourable breeding conditions for *Culex* mosquitoes will be increased by a greater use of wastewater for expanding agricultural purposes.

Enteric infection hazards

The hazards underlying enteric infections are the pathogenic organisms that cause them. These may be viruses, bacteria or protozoa. The resulting gastrointestinal infections, generically referred to as diarrhoeal diseases, are widespread in the Region. The disease burden they cause in the Region is estimated at 8 661 000 disability-adjusted life years (DALYs) lost [18], i.e. 14% of the global estimate (with, in comparison, 8% of the world population living in the countries of the Region).

The two major enteric diseases of viral origin are hepatitis A and poliomyelitis. Fortunately, most of the populations in the Region have a strong natural immunity against hepatitis A, and a large percentage of children have been vaccinated against poliomyelitis, thus substantially limiting the risk.

The two major protozoans causing enteric infections are *Giardia lamblia* (giardiasis) and *Entamoeba histolyticum* (amoebiasis). Giardiasis is relatively uncommon in the Region, but amoebiasis is widespread and is usually transmitted through vegetables grown on fields irrigated with untreated wastewater and not washed and/or cooked before consumption.

Bacterial enteric infections are numerous and range from salmonellosis and shigellosis (both transmitted most frequently through contaminated food) to typhoid fever and cholera (transmitted most frequently through contaminated drinking-water). The urban drinking-water supply is reliable and safe in most big cities, but rural populations may have to rely for their drinking-water needs on shallow wells or springs. Their drinking-water is therefore frequently subject to contamination by sewage, human excreta or other sources of infective material at any point between collection and consumption. As a result, the burden of enteric infections is greatest in rural and periurban populations. Lack of adequate sanitation further exacerbates the risk of exposure to these infections, through contamination of food and water.

Respiratory infection hazards

Acute respiratory infections are a very significant cause of child mortality and morbidity in the Region. Environmental risk factors for acute respiratory infection are poor housing, overcrowding of dwellings, poor heating when winters are exceptionally cold, and indoor and outdoor air pollution. These environmental risk factors, combined with malnutrition, facilitate the spread of tuberculosis, which is on the increase in many countries of the Region.

There is another type of acute respiratory infection, affecting mostly middle-aged men, which is transmitted through droplets emitted from poorly maintained air-conditioning systems or domestic warm water networks inside public buildings, such as hospitals or international hotels, and causes acute pneumonia called legionellosis. In the overall public health picture, the disease is marginal, but when an outbreak occurs, its mortality rate rapidly catches media attention, with detrimental economic consequences.

Chronic respiratory disease hazards

Chronic respiratory diseases are linked to indoor and outdoor air pollution. The genesis of these chronic respiratory diseases requires high levels of long-term human exposure, which is found among unprotected workers in mines, quarries and other specific industries, but not among the general population. Chronic respiratory diseases, such as pneumoconiosis, silicosis or fibrosis, are commonly found among miners and industrial workers in the Region.

Chemical hazards

Chemical poisonings occur in homes as a result of mishandling of chemical consumer products, such as cleaning media, cosmetic and pharmaceutical products, pesticides and so on. Chemical poisoning also occurs among workers in industries and handicraft workshops. Unprotected agricultural workers, in particular, may be exposed to important risks of acute pesticide poisoning.

Current levels of air, water and soil pollution by toxic chemicals are not sufficiently high in the Region to be an acute health hazard to its human populations. Introduction of new industries and also in case of a major industrial accident, the exposure of neighboring populations may, however, reach significant risk levels. Another risk in the Region is constituted by chemical poisoning through the consumption of unsafe food. A major accident of massive human intoxication by mercury compounds happened in Iraq in the 1970s, when rural populations mistakenly ate seeds that had been treated with a mercurial fungicide.

Carcinogenic hazards

Chemical poisoning is a problem only in case of high levels of exposure during a relatively short period; carcinogenic effects may appear as a result of long-term exposure to relatively small doses of carcinogenic chemicals or radiation. Relatively speaking, cancer is not the major cause of mortality as it is in some other regions, but it is an important cause of hospitalization. It is crucial that the general population be protected against excessive exposure to carcinogens. Those carcinogens may be found in consumer products such as tobacco, but they are usually chemicals emitted from industrial processes, which find their way to urban air, drinking-water or food. Ionizing radiation is carcinogenic, too, and exposure risks may be significantly high around nuclear plants.

High levels of ionizing radiation, coming from radon gas, may be found inside underground mines, especially when the bedrock is crystalline. Phosphate deposits and gypsum may also produce a significant amount of radiation as a by-product. No data are available, however, on the possible epidemiological impact of exposure to increased levels of radiation.

Hazards related to the depletion of good quality freshwater resources

Water is a scarce resource in most of the Region, and therefore any wastage of good quality fresh water will not only be an economic loss, but also a threat to human health. Freshwater resources are jeopardized through pollution of springs, streams, rivers, lakes and aquifers, or through the process of salinization resulting from excessive pumping of underground waters or from lack of proper drainage in irrigated areas. The pressure on freshwater resources comes mainly from agriculture, and different options to reduce this pressure (ranging from important water-intensive food products from outside the Region, to the use of wastewater for irrigation and the deployment of irrigation technologies aimed at saving water) should all be considered for their potential health impacts and health opportunities.

Underground water replenishment and water pollution prevention should be top priorities of governments in the Region.

Hazards related to the loss of good agricultural lands and/or fisheries depletion

Most countries of the Region suffer from a food production deficit, and any major loss of good agricultural land may threaten food security and undermine the nutritional status of the population. Agricultural land may be lost due to unplanned urbanization, construction of major reservoirs, or major transport infrastructures.

In a few countries, fisheries contribute significantly to the dietary protein component. Coastal and seawater pollution may have detrimental effects on fish nurseries and can lead to drastic reductions in fish stocks.

Types of projects and main environmental health impacts associated with them

This section is intended to provide guidance for the process of screening some of the major development projects that may have significant environmental health impacts, and for which a full EHIA may be needed. It was written with public health specialists in mind, who may require further information on project characteristics that are relevant from a health perspective.

Large reservoirs

Large reservoirs are developed for a range of purposes: drinking-water supply (especially for urban centres), irrigated agriculture and hydropower generation. Most frequently, they are multipurpose. The health impacts related to the construction of a dam and the creation of a man-made lake can be numerous, and depend on several characteristics of the reservoir [3,19]. The creation of a large water body in the arid and semi-arid conditions that prevail in the Region will have dramatic ecological consequences. The new land–water interface is the place where productive ecosystems are created; depending on the local terrain, this shoreline may vary considerably in length in relation to the reservoir's surface. Draw-down regimes will determine variation in shore length over time, and shores may be steep or shallow. The ecology of the reservoir itself will undergo rapid changes before it reaches a new steady state after about 15 years. Early on, organic matter may result in eutrophication; this may be maintained if major agricultural development takes place along the shores causing run-off of fertilizer. Toxic algal blooms may be a serious health hazard.

Human migration induced by a new reservoir adds to the complexity of possible health impacts. Furthermore, downstream effects on the water regime (for example, the interruption of seasonal flooding of the plains related to rainfall patterns) also need to be taken into account. Most large reservoirs are unique and require their individual EHIA.

The development of many small dams in a region may have an equal or even more pronounced impact on health, because of cumulative effects. In such a case, a strategic EHIA should address possible health implications.

While projects of this type may have many positive impacts because they increase freshwater availability, they may adversely affect the health of vulnerable communities if they are poorly planned. In brief, they may have the following negative health impacts:

- an increase of waterborne diseases if no water supply and sanitation facilities are created for communities along the shoreline and downstream of the dam;
- an increase in water-related vector-borne diseases because of the creation of suitable habitats for the propagation of disease vectors;
- an increase in water-based diseases (in particular schistosomiasis) whenever sanitation is inadequate and more intense water contact patterns occur;
- malnutrition caused by the loss of a large amount of good agricultural land or changes in the downstream water regime;
- loss of water quality through eutrophication and toxic effects of certain algal blooms.

Several other phenomena related to large reservoirs may have important health implications. At the construction phase the incidence of HIV/AIDS and other sexually transmitted infections may significantly increase. When a reservoir is invaded by aquatic weeds, excessive evaporation may significantly reduce the available water quantity. In some areas, the creation of large reservoirs has been accompanied by increased seismic activity or freak extreme weather patterns.

Examples

Lake Nasser, created by the construction of the new Aswan Dam in the Nile, has a total area of around 1200 km^2. Annual evaporation losses are estimated at an amount of 216 million cubic metres; other losses include that of good agricultural land and sediments trapped in the lake, which can no longer contribute to the fertilization of the downstream lands and which have also affected fisheries in the Mediterranean near the mouth of the river.

No serious direct health impacts have been recorded, however, probably because the Egyptian health services have extensive experience in schistosomiasis control, and have been able to prevent any expansion of this endemic disease. In addition, the positive impacts of Lake Nasser on Egyptian economic development are recognized as having contributed to many aspects of social development, including public health.

In Morocco, a new reservoir on the Ouerrha river was created to provide drinking-water for urban centres and for agricultural production purposes. An environmental impact assessment was implemented in accordance with Moroccan legislation. In the framework of this study, the Environmental Health unit of the Moroccan Ministry of Health carried out an EHIA.

The EHIA showed that this project had the potential to significantly increase malaria incidence in the neighbouring rural area. In response, mitigation measures were designed and implemented, including improved vector surveillance and control and strengthened case detection and treatment. While the choice of typically health sector-confined interventions reflects a rather conservative approach to the problem, it should be recognized that, since this reservoir has become operational, the measures have been successful and no significant increase of malaria incidence in the area has so far been observed.

Major irrigation schemes

Irrigated agriculture contributes importantly to food security in the Region. The introduction of irrigation in the climate conditions of the Region results in dramatic ecological changes with important human health dimensions. The most direct health impacts originate from the increase of mosquito and snail populations, with the resulting increase in malaria and schistosomiasis transmission. Leptospirosis, a bacterial zoonosis with rodent host species, is another important infectious disease risk. Different types of irrigation carry different types of risks: surface irrigation, with its extensive canal systems, frequently lacks sufficient drainage and the tendency towards excessive water intake creates more important risks than overhead (sprinkler) or drip irrigation. The latter also has important water saving aspects. Managing water better in surface irrigation schemes, through improved infrastructure, water management incentives and innovative techniques, such as surge irrigation, can help reduce risks. Tiffen [14] and Birley [16] describe the intersectoral planning process and the impact assessment and mitigation measures for irrigation schemes, respectively.

In addition to these direct health impacts, irrigation schemes are often accompanied by increased chemical inputs. The various health risks related to the use of pesticides and fertilizers are therefore also important. Poorly designed agricultural irrigation schemes may result in massive losses of good agricultural lands through salinization, if drainage is inadequate, and this, in turn, may have dire consequences for the nutritional status of local communities. A shift from subsistence to cash crop farming, often induced by irrigation development, can have similar effects on the local nutritional status. On the positive side, irrigation development is usually accompanied by infrastructural and service improvements, such as roads and electrification, with their concomitant health benefits. Surprisingly, however, irrigation schemes continue to be constructed that do not have an adequate drinking-water supply component.

Example

The Gezira development, a large-scale agricultural development project undertaken during colonial times in the Gezira area of Sudan, resulted in a major double epidemic of malaria and schistosomiasis, eventually resulting in the endemicity of both diseases. This is probably the worse public health disaster on record in Sudan. At the time, EHIA and EIA had not been developed. In the last few years, the Government of Sudan has made extensive efforts to address environmental health impacts and respond to them through safeguards and mitigation measures.

Treated sewage use for irrigated agriculture

In the water-scarce Eastern Mediterranean Region, wastewater is an important resource. WHO has norms and standards for its safe use in agriculture and aquaculture [20,21]. The level of risk is related to the extent of treatment of the wastewater before use. Various communities are at risk, with microbiological hazards including bacterial and viral pathogens, eggs of intestinal helminths (worms) and a range of chemical pollutants, including heavy metals. In the disposal of wastewater, another range of hazards and risks are of importance. There may be an impact on unconfined aquifers and on the shallow wells from which rural populations take their drinking-water.

Cement and phosphate plants and quarries

Cement and phosphate plants produce large emissions of dust. Populations living downwind of the plant stack will breathe in high levels of dust, and are therefore exposed to hazards that may lead to chronic respiratory diseases. Dusty air also increases the seriousness of infectious respiratory diseases, as well as of eye diseases. Mineral extraction is an important economic activity in many countries of the Region. The main health impacts of quarries include injuries among workers, and chronic respiratory diseases resulting from workers' excessive exposure to mineral dust. Quarries have little health impacts outside the work environment unless they are located adjacent to populated areas.

Oil production, oil refineries and petrochemical industries

The oil resources in the Region are among the most important in the world, and particularly in the Gulf Cooperation Council countries there is extensive industrial infrastructure for extraction, transport and processing. Without proper safeguards, the various components and activities of this industry may result in major pollution, with significant public health consequences. Well-drilling uses lubricant sludge that contains many hazardous chemicals. Around wells there is leakage of this sludge, and also leakage of oil. Such leakage may pollute underground water resources, lakes and coastal waters. Leakage of oil and sludge may also pollute soils, destroying their agricultural production capacity. This impact is minimal, however, wherever oilfields are located in the desert.

Oil transportation may also be a source of leakage and spills that can pollute fresh water, agricultural lands, rangelands, coastal areas and the sea. Coastal pollution may have a detrimental impact on fish nurseries and marine ecology, and may affect the nutritional status of local communities.

The entire production chain, from extraction, transportation to refining, is at high risk of fires and explosions. Its direct health impacts are therefore related to injuries and burns among workers and the neighbouring population; its indirect health impacts result from contamination of fresh water and loss of food production assets.

In addition, oil refining and petrochemical industries emit significant quantities of toxic chemicals into the air, water and soil. Through inhalation or ingestion, those chemicals may be absorbed by the populations living around the plants, and also the unprotected workers inside the plants. Among the chemicals worth noting are poly-cyclic aromatic hydrocarbons (PAH), which are suspected to be carcinogenic. Some blends of oil (for example, oil from the Caucasian area) have a high content of PAH, other blends of oil (for example, the so-called Arabian light) have a low content. Excessive exposure of the surrounding populations to PAH emissions creates a risk of increased cancer incidence. Available statistics show mainly the casualties resulting from oil fires and explosions. In many instances, monitoring by the health services lacks sufficient sensitivity to pick up increases in cancer prevalence around oil refineries or petrochemical plants, while in other places mortality and morbidity caused by infectious diseases is a masking factor.

Chemical industries

The oil industry is only one branch among the large family of chemical industries. The most common chemical industries in the Region, other than the petrochemical industry, include the manufacturing of fertilizers, pesticides, paints and dyes. All chemical industries are liable to accidents and explosions. In the case of large-scale industrial explosions, the neighbouring population may be badly affected. This is why chemical industries must be located as far away as possible from human settlements, inside especially engineered industrial parks, and illegal urbanization around the plants must be prevented. In addition, all chemical industries are potential sources of toxic chemical emissions in air, water and soil.

Among the most hazardous industries are pesticide-manufacturing plants, as they deal with products which affect basic biological mechanisms.

Steelworks and other metal industries

Inside metallurgic industries workers are exposed to hazards that imply a high risk of injury, to excessive noise and heat, and to various toxic chemicals, fumes and heavy metals. Wherever those industries are not located in specially designed industrial parks, the surrounding population may also be at risk.

Actually steelworks do not emit large amounts of toxic metals, but non-ferrous metal industries do emit such toxic particulates. Lead smelting leads to the emission of lead dust, zinc smelting to the emission of cadmium, and aluminum smelting to the emission of fluorine. Galvanic industries release cyanide in wastewater. Such emissions have an impact on the health of surrounding populations among which intoxication cases may eventually be observed.

Seawater desalinization plants

Two different processes to desalinate water exist: the flash–distillation process which is a thermal process for which energy consumption is in relation to the volume of water treated but not of the amount of salt removed; and the reverse osmosis process which is a membrane process for which energy consumption is related to the amount of salt removed, but not of the amount of water treated. Reverse osmosis is the most efficient process to treat brackish water, but flash–distillation is the best to treat seawater with a high salt content, as is the case for the Red Sea, or the waters of the Persian Gulf.

The by-product of both processes is a large amount of brine, which has to be disposed of and is generally discharged into the sea. Another problem has its origin in the use of anti-fouling products to protect pipes from excessive invasion of marine organisms, and of paints to protect those pipes against corrosion. Brine discharge, in addition to leakage of anti-fouling and anti-corrosion products, has detrimental impacts on marine life, and especially on fish. Therefore, poorly planned seawater desalination plants may have a detrimental impact on fish resources and, consequently, on the nutritional and overall economic status of local fishing communities.

Phosphate mining and other mines

Mining to exploit mineral resources can be done either through digging in the open air, or through underground burrows. The main impacts are injuries among miners, followed by chronic respiratory diseases due to inhalation of dust, and sometimes lung cancer due to radon exposure if underground mining take place, as small amounts of uranium are often part of phosphate rock layers.

If mining is performed in the open air, neighbouring populations are exposed to mineral dust and possibly to particles loaded with heavy metals. Lead will come from lead mining, cadmium from zinc mining, and mercury emissions may come from the use of mercury to extract some precious metals, such as gold or silver. Wherever mining is performed underground, however, exposure levels of the neighbouring populations will be significantly lower. If a mine is located inside a narrow mountain valley, dust concentration in the vicinity of the mine will be significantly higher than in a plain setting, due to the lack of atmospheric dispersion.

Phosphate mining usually takes place in the open air and is a major dust producer, creating a risk of chronic respiratory diseases and also a risk of eye diseases; but the main problems come from two by-products often found inside phosphate deposits, fluorine and uranium. A high prevalence of fluorosis can be observed among populations living around phosphate mines, but no significant increases in the incidence of cancers, such as leukemia, have been reported, despite significant levels of uranium inside phosphate deposits.

Examples

Saturnism, i.e. lead intoxication, is common among lead miners but usually does not affect the miners' families. However, at least one case was recorded in eastern Morocco, where saturnism was diagnosed among members of miners' families living close to a lead mine. In central Morocco, where large-scale phosphate mining is practised, high prevalence of tooth fluorosis is commonly recorded among children, but the potential health impact of uranium by-products has not been demonstrated.

Fossil-fuel fired power plants

The main impact of thermal power plants is air pollution by SO_2, NO_x and particulates. This pollution has negative impacts on the lung functions of the population living in the vicinity of the plant. The release of cooling water of these plants into water bodies results in thermal pollution, an important environmental impact. In the Eastern Mediterranean Region, many power plants are sited on the coast and use seawater for cooling purposes. An excessive increase of coastal water temperature may be detrimental to local marine life and may drastically deplete fish stocks.

Major transportation infrastructures, airports and highways

When located inside agricultural lands, transport infrastructures will lead to the loss of large amounts of scarce agricultural land and reduce the national capacity to produce food. Such infrastructures also become sources of noise and air pollution. The negative impacts of these types of nuisance on human beings are, however, only significant in nearby urban areas. There is extensive experience and knowledge of the health impacts of airplane noise on those living in the flight path areas around airports. High blood pressure is one of the key health effects.

Other than accident and injury, one of the main health impacts of transport infrastructures is that they facilitate the circulation of pathogenic germs. Their introduction into areas where the local population lacks natural or acquired immunity may cause major infectious disease outbreaks.

Liquid or solid waste disposal facilities

The building of waste disposal facilities is basically an asset for public health as it decreases pollution of land and waters. However, improperly planned facilities may have negative impacts overriding their positive ones. For example, a waste incinerator located inside an urban area may be a major source of air pollution for this area. A poorly operated composting plant is a major source of unpleasant smells. A sanitary landfill located too close to an urban area may be a source of infections and nuisances, and it will attract scavengers, who will be exposed to the worst possible occupational conditions.

Wastewater treatment plants may create health risks when the treatment is inefficient, or when unsafe reuse of the effluent takes place. Industrial wastewater includes toxic compounds and therefore should not be discharged in municipal sewers without prior chemical neutralization. In some countries of the Region, industrial wastewater is stored in large ponds. In such cases, the ponds should be effectively fenced, as there are a number of reported cases of children having drowned in these ponds.

Hazards and vulnerability

Even at the screening stage, some understanding of the mechanisms that link hazards to specific community groups and that underlie the translation from changes in environmental health determinants into health risks is essential. This section singles out three important areas: infection pathways, chemical exposure and the context of natural resources development.

Assessment of infection risks

Pathogens have biologically evolved to survive inside the human body or in an environment similar to that of the human body. Generally, pathogens cannot survive over extended periods of time under extreme temperatures or with a total lack of water. The eggs of many intestinal helminths (worms) are exceptional in terms of survival under adverse conditions. Many human pathogens, though not all, may, however, survive in their adult stage in the body of other warm-blooded animals; these are referred to as reservoirs. Some human parasites may require that part of their biological life-cycle take place inside the body of an animal. If an animal (for example, an aquatic snail) plays a strictly passive role of hosting the parasite, it is called an intermediate host. A vector, on the contrary, not only provides the environment for life-cycle development of a pathogen, but it also plays an active role in transmission usually through biting (e.g. insects). Diseases for which there is an animal reservoir are called zoonoses, and diseases for which intermediate hosts or vectors play a role in the transmission cycle are referred to as vector-borne diseases. They all have in common that they are closely linked to specific ecological conditions that are suitable for the animal reservoirs, intermediate hosts or vectors. Environmental management approaches to control them aim at modifying those conditions permanently or temporarily.

Humans become infected by microbial pathogens through inhalation of viruses or bacteria present in droplets or aerosols, through ingestion of contaminated food or water, through penetration of the skin by insects or parasites, or through bites of animals or stings of insects. The "infective dose" is specific to each pathogen, and is the minimum adequate dose to allow its further multiplication in the human host that eventually leads to the clinical symptoms.

The human immune system provides some level of innate resistance, newborn babies acquire antibodies from their mother and once the immune system develops, children start to develop acquired immunity against the most common microbes with which they are in contact. Vaccination is the artificial way to create individual immunity against specific microbes, usually viruses. Immunity against human pathogens is weakened among the elderly, and among especially vulnerable groups (e.g. those undergoing certain drug therapies and those infected with HIV/AIDS). Malnutrition renders young children especially sensitive to infections, and some infections (such as malaria) may suppress the immune system and allow normally mildly pathogenic microbes to turn virulent. A population is vulnerable to infection and an epidemic may develop if it lacks immunity against this specific infection. This is most often seen when communities move from a non-malarious to a malarious area.

The vulnerability of a population also depends on the effectiveness of the local health services. Effective health systems will be able to detect an epidemic risk at an early stage. Corrective actions may be initiated immediately, through identification, isolation and treatment of cases. In most instances, this will limit and control the outbreak. Pathogens include viruses, bacteria, and two kinds of parasites: protozoa and worms. Viruses cannot survive for long outside a living cell, and they are not sensitive to antibiotics, but vaccines are available to protect against the most common viruses. There are many kinds of pathogenic bacteria, and the standard method of treating bacterial infections is through the use of antibiotics. Resistance to antibiotics is increasingly a problem. Parasites have complex life-cycles, no vaccines to protect against them exist and they often show molecular strategies to escape from the host's immune response. Drug resistance is a growing problem, as is the case with malaria.

Four species of protozoan parasites, all belonging to the genus *Plasmodium*, cause malaria in humans. These parasites rely on a transition through the *Anopheles* mosquito as part of their life-cycle for sexual reproduction and development. *Anopheles* larvae develop in clean bodies of fresh water and the female mosquito needs a blood meal prior to reproduction. The larval ecology of anophelines varies, from sunlit pools, to slowly moving streams, to shaded water collections in forests and urban, man-made water collections. The adult mosquito may show a variety of biting and resting behaviours that are also important for the disease ecology. The mosquito becomes infected through biting infected humans, and the parasite goes through a physiological change inside the mosquito to end up as infective larvae in the mosquito's salivary glands. A warm and humid climate is conducive to the development of mosquitoes and of the parasite. The arid areas of the Eastern Mediterranean Region are, therefore, at a lesser risk of malaria transmission.

Schistosomiasis or bilharzia is caused by blood flukes of the genus *Schistosoma*, worms that live in pairs in human blood vessels, where they reproduce and lay eggs. The passage of eggs through the tissues of the intestines or bladder cause the pathogenic effect. The eggs are excreted with urine or stool (depending on the *Schistosoma* species) and, in an aquatic environment, they hatch to release larvae which infest snails and develop, inside the snail, to free swimming infective larvae called cercariae; there may penetrate the human body through the skin. This complex life-cycle has various stages at which control interventions are feasible.

Protozoans of the genus *Leishmania* survive in host reservoirs, rural wild rodents of several species, and are transmitted by their vector, sandflies of the genus *Phlebotomus*. Any environmental change that creates conditions favourable to the propagation of rodents or of sandflies, increases the risk of *Leishmania* transmission. The resulting disease can be of a visceral form, affecting internal organs, usually with a high mortality rate, or of a cutaneous form, causing skin lesions, such as the Aleppo sore. This depends on the *Leishmania* species involved.

These three parasitic diseases are mainly found in rural areas. In addition to the vector species-related ecological determinants, there are also important social determinants, with poverty being the main one. Malaria and leishmaniasis are rapidly developing, acute diseases, while schistosomiasis is a slowly developing, chronic debilitating illness.

Chemical behaviour in the environment

Industrial activities generate pollutants which are usually discharged in the environment as atmospheric emissions or as liquid or solid waste discharges. Human beings may absorb pollutants which are included in the air they breathe, the water they drink or the food they eat, without taking into account the limited number of pollutants that may cross the skin barrier directly. The exposure pathways of pollutants and their absorption by humans are associated with their physicochemical characteristics. They will concentrate preferably in specific media with which they have links. For example, volatile chemicals will disperse in the air, water soluble chemicals will concentrate in any water they may reach, chemicals with high capacity of adsorption will concentrate in soils, and more specifically in soils with organic matter.

After having reached their favourite medium, chemicals may undergo two kinds of processes: transformation and/or concentration. Through biochemical transformations a chemical will be changed in two or several metabolites, usually less offensive, but sometimes more offensive than the original compound. For example, metallic mercury is not absorbed in the human metabolic system, but through biological transformation, specific bacteria may change metallic mercury into methyl-mercury which can be absorbed by humans and is a deadly poison.

Physical concentration takes place in accordance to respective density and solubility. For example, heavy particulates from an atmospheric emission will sediment quickly on the soil and accumulate with time; water-soluble products will concentrate in water bodies; fat-soluble chemicals eventually fall down on pasture and may be recycled by animals feeding on those pastures, and so accordingly will concentrate in animal fat. Biological concentration of chemicals may also take place along the food-chain, the concentrations growing from prey to predator. Some persistent pollutants of an organic nature may not only accumulate in the food-chain, but also concentrate in specific regions of the world with a greater inertia. The highest concentrations of persistent organic pollutants (POPs) are found in the ice of glaciers and in the polar ice caps.

When significant emissions of a specific toxic chemical from any project are identified, there is a need to characterize this chemical using the "chemical safety data sheets", available from the IRPTC (International Registry of Potentially Toxic Chemicals), which is jointly operated by the United Nations Environment Programme/World Health Organization/Food and Agriculture Organization of the United Nations and the International Labour Organization and may be contacted through the Programme on Chemical Safety at WHO, Geneva (www.who.int/ipcs/en). The EHIA terms of reference may refer to specific datasheets for the consultants to follow up.

The absorbed doses may be computed on the basis of the potential concentration of pollutant, multiplied by the quantity of drink or food absorbed daily. The WHO/FAO *Codex Alimentarius* lists, for the more commonly used chemicals, the maximum daily intake which does not affect human health. If those levels are trespassed, detrimental impacts on the health of sensitive individuals may be observed and those ill-health impacts will augment with increasing average absorbed doses. Again, reference to the relevant dose–response curves can be made in the EHIA terms of reference or in an annex to the terms of reference. Consultants should be requested, however, to cover, in their EHIA, the human toxicity aspects of a comprehensive range of chemicals that are ·relevant in relation to the proposed project.

When toxicity only is involved (i.e. when the chemical is a poison), toxicologists can recognize that there is a non-effect level below which no ill-health impacts will take place. But when the chemical is a carcinogen, there is no non-effect level, as the risk will be proportional to the cumulative absorbed dose. The same proportionality to the cumulative absorbed dose applies to exposure to ionizing radiation, which is also carcinogenic.

Contrary to biological pathogens, toxic chemicals do not multiply, they may only be transformed or concentrated. This facilitates their control.

Social determinants and population vulnerability

The risks related to many health hazards are associated with a complex mixture of environmental and social determinants. Malnutrition is probably the most clearcut example where the social determinants of health are singularly important. The vulnerability of population groups to malnutrition is closely linked to their social characteristics.

Any significant loss of basic natural resources (land and water) is an indirect threat for public health in terms of nutritional status. Quantity and balance are critical elements of a healthy diet. The social determinants that influence nutrition include, first of all, poverty, but also equity, gender, education levels and the various social and economic incentives to use natural resources in alternative ways.

Food security in the Region depends significantly on the policies of governments to provide subsidies for basic staple foods. Many of these need to be imported and will in theory be more expensive than locally produced food. Yet trade tariffs, taxes and subsidies may change this picture. For example, governments will want to promote crops that are less reliant on water, in line with the generalized water scarcity.

Seemingly unrelated policies in the water sector may also have unforeseen effects on health; for example, the promotion of small-scale hydropower projects has a great potential to reduce the burden of acute respiratory diseases, as it reverses the use of fuels that cause indoor air pollution.

Many issues of ill-health are related to specific occupations, and this is another, partially socially determined health burden. Fishing communities will be vulnerable to schistosomiasis, agriculturalists run the risk of exposure to pesticides and their residues, and miners are exposed to toxic fumes.

At specific stages of a project, social conditions may arise that carry specific health risks. The influx of construction workers in a dam project carries not only the risk of sexually transmitted infection, but also of substance abuse.

As stated at the beginning of this chapter, screening of projects is mainly a desk exercise. In many countries there will be clearly defined criteria geared towards the screening of projects for the need of environmental assessments. These can be expanded to take health issues into account. Yet the complexity of many health issues often requires more than the simple ticking of boxes on a screening checklist. It is important to refer to well-documented historic case studies and to investigate, at least superficially, infection and exposure pathways that are realistically feasible in a setting of development induced change. This will strengthen the decision-making on whether or not to carry out an EHIA, and in the event the answer to that question is affirmative, it allows for more comprehensive and targeted terms of reference for the consultants from whom the EHIA will be commissioned.

Chapter 4
Elements and methods to carry out EHIA studies

> This chapter elaborates on the actual commissioning of environmental health impact assessments. The criteria contained in the government's screening policy, as outlined in Chapter 1, will lead to a decision on whether or not a project requires an EHIA.
>
> Once this has been determined and affirmed, the project proponent has the responsibility to implement the EHIA or to contract it out to a specialized consultant. To ensure that health and environmental impacts are comprehensively and adequately covered, the government agency in charge of project licensing provides a framework for the EHIA in the form of terms of reference.
>
> In this chapter the structural elements of the terms of reference are presented in a logical sequence. It proposes methods to deal with the terms of reference elements and to synthesize the outcome of each element into a final, comprehensive assessment. The terms of reference framework also provides the starting point for the independent appraisal of the EHIA report. The next chapter links the elements presented here to the criteria and procedures of the quality control component of the excercise.

Procedure

One option to ensure an accurate and efficient assessment of the health impact of development policies, programmes or projects is to combine it with environmental impact assessment, so that EIA becomes EHIA. The ready-made tool of environmental impact assessment provides an appropriate and time-tested procedural framework for the assessment of health impacts. Many countries in the Eastern Mediterranean Region have already established an EIA unit or environmental protection agency and given it statutory duties to examine new projects for their environmental impacts. Yet, whereas EIA procedures may well exist, they are not always given serious attention. Expanding existing EIA procedures into EHIA offers good opportunities to detect and correct generic weaknesses and shortcomings of impact assessment at large.

Reference to health in EIAs has tended to be limited. The limitations are twofold. First, the conventional concepts of health, outside but often also within the health sector, are mainly sectoral in nature. As a result, EIAs consider the protection and promotion of health to be exclusively within the remit of the health sector. Their recommendations therefore seldom address design and operational alternatives to reduce health risks. Most frequently they focus on strengthening health sector functions in response to adverse health impacts.

Secondly, the health issue most commonly included in EIAs relates to the toxic effects of pollution. This reflects key concerns of industrialized countries, where EIA was conceived in the 1960s and 1970s. In the context of industrialization, transport and traffic expansion and the construction of thermal power plants and dams, this type of impact has received a lot of attention and much is known about it. Dose–response curves allow for a semi-quantitative risk evaluation. Other types of health impacts, such as occupational injury, mental health problems and even communicable diseases, have, for a long time, remained in the shadow of pollution-related health issues. Upgrading EIA to a proper EHIA will make it necessary to add a statutory requirement to assess health as a cross-cutting issue in development. This calls for three important steps to be taken.

- The role and responsibilities of the Ministry of Health in all critical steps of the assessment procedure must be defined and formalized (see Chapter 1).
- Based on the initial screening, health elements must be added specifically to the terms of reference that set the framework for the impact assessment commissioned from consultants. These elements must emphasize the intersectoral nature of health issues and the need to address health comprehensively (see Chapter 2).
- An independent mechanism for appraising completed health impact assessments must be established to determine their adequacy.

Project proponents (who may be government officers from other sectors or private sector entrepreneurs) will generally not undertake an assessment themselves, as they have neither the time nor the training. Instead, they will contract the task out to a consultant and then manage the consultant's outputs. It is crucial to ensure that the consultant who undertakes the assessment has full access to all relevant project documentation, all relevant key informants and all health statistics. Experience has shown that the technical know-how and skills of a physician or clinician usually do not meet the needs of an EHIA adequately. A generalist with a background in public health, human ecology and/or environmental health best fits the desired profile. In addition to a broad public health background, the consultant should also be a capable communicator and a team leader who can delegate subtasks to, preferably local, experts.

It is in principle correct to place health impact assessment under the jurisdiction of the Ministry of Health's Environmental Health Department and its staff of environmental health officers, as they have the right background and training. Unfortunately, environmental health units, if existing as separate entities at all, have always been in the margins of the health sector. They have been further weakened in recent years in the context of government decentralization and many environmental health workers have been dispersed either to district level or to units in other public sectors. In addition, many conflicting or overlapping laws cover the statutory duties and essential functions of environmental health officers, while there are also gaps in their jurisdiction. In most countries of the Region, environmental health officers have not been trained in health impact assessment and so lack the capability to participate and contribute to the process.

In any event, the establishment of EHIA policies, procedures and methods always requires, as a first step, capacity-building within the health sector, so it can effectively collaborate with the environmental authorities and respond to the needs of the development sectors and project proponents. WHO can provide modules, materials and technical support for the organization of a national start-up workshop for the health sector, and for the creation of a structure within the health sector that will support the procedures ensuring optimal performance of essential health impact assessment functions at the different administrative levels.

Method

With policies, structures and procedures in place, the stage is set to routinely undertake environmental health impact assessments. A simple, rapid and structured method is required. It must include all the relevant elements and its results must be presented in a logical and consistent manner.

Gathering data

There are two main methods available of gathering data in support of an EHIA. These are: key informant interview and literature review (see below). It is important to keep a balance between the two, and not just to collect the data, but also analyse them. Inevitably, there will be important gaps in the datasets and these will have to be filled by assumptions. This is appropriate, provided all the assumptions are clearly stated, so the reader is free to agree or disagree. The literature review will draw on published and unpublished papers, reports and newspaper articles. The Internet is also a good data source. All data presented should be properly referenced and cited. There will rarely be time for proper collection of new scientific data or for epidemiological surveys, although social surveys of affected communities may be necessary and possible (see below). Large-scale projects may, however, require in addition a baseline survey to be used for further monitoring and surveillance.

The intensity of data gathering will be high in the early stages of any project, to facilitate proper design and to support economic feasibility studies, EIA and EHIA. Coordination is of the essence to minimize duplication of efforts and to ensure an optimal analysis of the association between different datasets. As yet unresolved constraints in such analyses relate to issues of scale and boundaries [22].

Sources of information

EHIA reports must always include a section describing the method or procedure followed in the collection of information, and the sources of information about a project and the project area, so that at the appraisal phase an informed conclusion can be reached about the reliability of the impact's knowledge base. Available information will often be incomplete, biased or uncertain. It will range in certainty from scientifically tested, through probable to speculative. It can be quantitative (in absolute terms or ranked in relative terms) or qualitative only. All evidence is valid as long as the assessment report is explicit about the assumptions applied and the uncertainties included. Possible sources of information include:

Government health statistics. Governments compile medical statistics based on the records of people seeking medical care from hospitals and health centres. Such data are sometimes inaccurate because of underreporting and lack of resources for adequate record keeping. Not all diseases are reportable. The data should, however, suggest which diseases are most common in a district, region or country and allow for them to be ranked. In the majority of countries of the Region, the most common causes of illness listed will be diarrhoea and respiratory disease.

In many countries, there are private as well as government medical facilities. People often prefer the private facilities because of low standards of government operated medical facilities. But private facilities do not report their statistics to government and this may be one important source of bias.

Knowledge is the currency of power and even in the statistical units of a health ministry it may, therefore, be difficult to obtain insight into data that are supposed to be in the public domain.

Key informant interview. The assessment will often be based on a series of interviews with key informants. Careful records should be kept about who was interviewed, when and where. These informants will include experts associated with the project and institutions that have a duty to protect human health. Examples may include transport officials, ministries responsible for labour, public works, irrigation, the environment, agriculture and industry.

There are many different units within a health ministry, including those responsible for environmental health. As ministries of health usually are severely underfunded and dominated by physicians, most of its resources are likely to be earmarked for curative medicine. Consequently, units of a more preventive nature, such as environmental health may have been neglected, run-down and their staff demoralized so that their value as sources of information may be far lower than expected.

Experts affiliated with academic institutions will have detailed knowledge of some aspects of a problem. For example, parasitologists may have conducted special surveys of the project community to determine the prevalence rate of particular infections, such as intestinal nematodes. These individuals may provide a relatively independent and unbiased view that can be compared to that of official statistics.

In any case, the interviews should be carried out covering a comprehensive range of people (professionals, working class, male, female, old, young). This process allows for the obtainment of more than one set of information to support and corroborate or to reject the conclusions and opinions of others.

Project documents. By the time an assessment is made, the project will have been through an identification, pre-feasibility and possibly feasibility phase. If the project is receiving external support there will be copious documents available that support the need and value of the proposal. These should detail the changes to the infrastructure that are planned together with the topography and other physical characteristics of the project site.

Literature review. The best information on the basis of which one can predict what will happen in a new project is the documented evidence of what has happened in similar projects in the same country or region. Information of this sort is often compiled by scientists and published in journals and books. It may also have been compiled in reports that have not been formally published. Grey literature is a valuable source of information but difficult to obtain. It is often stored in the libraries of consultancy companies, donor agencies, non-governmental organizations and UN institutions, such as WHO. There are also compilations of examples of the type of health impacts that may be relevant for each kind of project [23, 24]. An increasing amount of information is available on the Internet.

Procedural matters. In addition to sources of information relevant to the assessment method, there are sources of information about the procedures and policy context in which the assessment is being conducted.

Some donor agencies may have produced guidelines for the inclusion of health in their own impact assessment procedures. Examples include the Asian Development Bank [25] and the World Bank [17]. Some national governments, such as Australia [26], New Zealand [27] Canada [24], and the Philippines [28], have done the same. Other countries, such as the UK, have begun to establish national policies [29]. The European Union has established a policy requirement in the Maastricht Treaty [30].

Guidelines are also available to assist with the more detailed analysis of particular problems, such as vector-borne diseases associated with water resources development [16].

Scoping

The scope of the assessment, established through the preliminary desk exercise, must first be verified. This is accomplished through discussions with relevant experts, a review of existing documentation and, if strictly necessary, visits to the project site. It will confirm the geographical boundaries of the assessment and the number of years into the future over which health impacts are to be considered.

Geographical boundaries

The health impacts of a project may occur both inside and outside the boundaries of the project site. In the case of air and water pollution they may occur far downwind and downstream. In the case of health impacts with predominantly social determinants, they may occur in the distant homes of migrant labourers. They will certainly affect all the communities that live around the project site. In some cases transboundary impacts should be considered in the framework of existing international agreements. The spatial boundaries of an EIA and an EHIA may be different, depending on the location of affected communities, the distribution of population densities and human circulation patterns.

Temporal boundaries

Health impacts of any development project will vary considerably over the different project stages. The changes in health hazards and the vulnerable groups during the construction stage are likely to be very different from those occurring during the operational stage. For example, infrastructure projects requiring extensive construction will involve single male workers who live away from their families for considerable periods of time while earning good wages. Such a community attracts camp followers who sell food, drugs and sex. One of the consequences may be an epidemic of sexually transmitted infections (e.g. HIV/AIDS), which can also have a secondary impact on the health of mother and child populations once the workers return home. During the operational stage the worker community will be more settled. Health impacts may shift to accidents and injuries or to exposure to pesticides and pesticide residues. EHIA may stretch as far as decommissioning and post decommissioning of a project, but normally a balance is struck between the accuracy of the predictions (which will diminish the further the time horizon), and the resources available for the EHIA. As a rule of thumb, it is usually adequate to fix the end-point of the assessment to the conclusion of the early operation stage. By that time, a new steady state will have developed which the routine health services should be able to deal with.

Nevertheless, attention must be drawn to the fact that chemical or radioactive materials released during operational stages or even during the stages of construction or equipment

Environmental health impact assessment of development projects

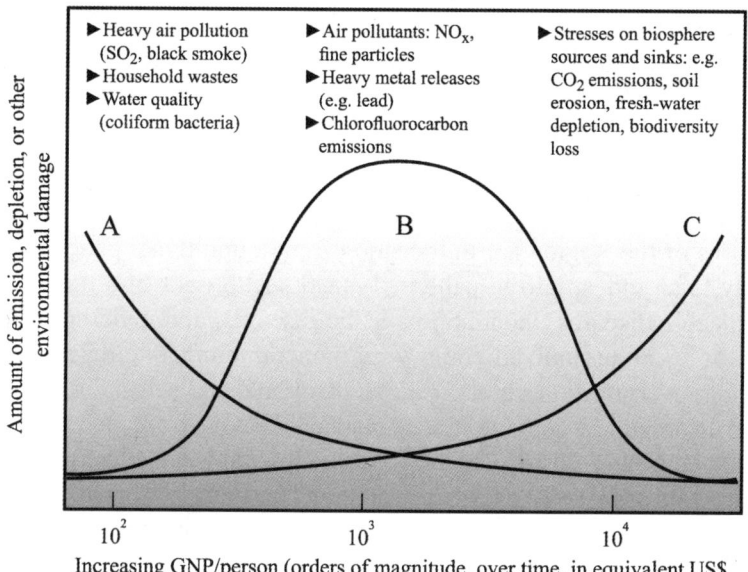

Figure 5. *The epidemiological transition from the rural to the urban setting: the descending line reflects the communicable disease risks, the ascending line the noncommunicable disease risks, in percentage points. The sum of both risks peaks for populations of periurban environments.*

Source: [31]

installation/testing may cause DNA changes that might put at jeopardy the health of future generations.

Health hazard identification

The recommended starting point of any EHIA is to make a list of all the possible health hazards that could be associated with the project under consideration. Consulting a standard reference [23] facilitates the production of such an inventory. Completing the list can be achieved by holding brainstorming sessions with a group of experts from different sectors. The hazards on the list can be organized into five main categories, with transmission exposure pathways and intervention options as key criteria:

- agents of communicable diseases (such as the malaria parasite);
- agents of noncommunicable diseases (such as a pesticide);
- agents or causes of physical injury (such as traffic and mechanical devices);
- causes of malnutrition (such as hunger);
- causes of psychosocial disorder (such as inequity or gender imbalance).

The assessment must seek to demonstrate plausibly how these hazards will be changed by the project. Impacts on human communities should also be considered, as well as the project's effect on social equity. The assessment should also help identify opportunities for health promotion created by the project.

Example

Many countries of the Region are in transition from a traditional pattern of morbidity and mortality to an industrialized pattern. Typical health risks of a traditional society are communicable diseases, including parasitic diseases, and undernutrition. Typical health risks of an industrialized country are noncommunicable diseases associated with poisoning; overnutrition; intentional, unintentional and self-induced injuries; and psychosocial disorders. As communities or individuals move from their rural homes into the urban and periurban environment, or from a traditional to an industrialized economy, the traditional health risks are expected to decline and the industrial health risks to increase. At the intermediate point, which may characterize many communities in countries of the Region, both kinds of risk may be present (see Figure 5). Thus communities may be afflicted with both tuberculosis associated with crowded living conditions and lung diseases associated with air pollution; or cholera associated with faecal contamination of water supplies and heavy metal intoxication associated with pollution by industrial wastes. Communities of this kind are often found in the periurban informal settlements that characterize many developing country cities. Such communities are often outside the jurisdiction of municipal authorities and are not provided with water supplies, sanitation or solid waste disposal. They frequently buy their water from vendors at extortionate prices and dispose of their waste indiscriminately. Informal settlements of this nature occur around cities in the Region. Experience elsewhere suggests that they cannot be effectively legislated against, bulldozed or ignored. It is necessary to bring them under the jurisdiction of a municipal authority and provide land tenure and services.

The traditional health risks tend to have a focus, obvious causality and low latency. For example, cholera results from drinking contaminated water or from eating salads grown with wastewater during the summer months. The industrial health risks tend to have less obvious causes and very long latencies, so that it is sometimes difficult to attribute a health outcome to a particular exposure event. For example, cancer may result from exposure to a set of carcinogens over 30 years. There are many exceptions, however; for example, the cause of traffic injury is immediately apparent.

In the case of traditional risks and some modern risks, health records, such as hospital admissions, can provide an indicator of changing health risk patterns. Since some modern health risks have long latency and complex causes, health data may not provide a useful indicator of changing risks. In these cases it is more useful to monitor and control likely causes, such as sources of pollution.

Exposed and vulnerable communities

All individuals affected by a project in any way will be exposed to its impacts. There are usually several different communities affected by a project, each made up of a number of community groups. Each community group will be exposed to different combinations of health hazards. So the next step is to identify the most vulnerable communities. Usually, these are the weakest and most vulnerable people, and if they are protected, then everybody will be protected. Poverty is the key determinant of vulnerability; families headed by single women make up another vulnerable group. According to the equity principle, it is advisable that the exposed communities share in the project benefits and that they are compensated for the risks they run involuntarily [15].

In fact, World Commission on Dams proposed five core values that need to be complied with to ensure a full knowledge and understanding of the benefits, impacts and risks of development projects (in the case of the World Commission on Dams, dams): equity, efficiency, participatory decision-making, sustainability and accountability. These same values can also be found in the impact assessment literature. Reconciling competing needs and entitlements in the context of development is, according to the World Commission on Dams, the single most important factor in conflict resolution. Recognizing rights and assessing risks in the project cycle offer a means of applying the core values to development decision-making. From the rights perspective, a proper impact assessment facilitates the identification of legitimate stakeholders and their rights and responsibilities. From the perspective of risk, a sound analysis will help distinguish those stakeholders who take and accept risks of development voluntarily and those who have risks imposed on them involuntarily. This helps determine which stakeholders are entitled to a place at the negotiating table, and forms a basis for an eventual programme of benefit sharing and compensation.

No project can be considered sustainable if it fails to determine the fears and concerns of affected communities and does not act upon them. Public participation in the EHIA process is therefore crucial. A local university social science department can be approached to carry out a social survey. The issues to address, through semi-structured interviews, focus group discussions and open questions, are the risk factors identified during the assessment (see Table 1) and their components, as well as community perceptions and how these relate to reality. Table 1 shows the exposed communities associated with a wastewater reuse project, together with their potential exposure to six excreta-related disease categories.

Latency and persistence are the distinguishing features of these six excreta-related disease categories. Transmission entry points are also different (oral or through the skin). Latency refers to the period between the moment of excretion and the moment the pathogen becomes infectious. Persistence is a measure of the viability of a pathogen

Table 1. Example of community exposure to excreta-related diseases

Communities	Hepatitis	Typhoid, cholera	Ascariasis	Hookworm infection	Tapeworm infection	Schisto-somiasis
Members of rural households	*	*	*	*		*
Sewage plant workers	*	*	*	*		
Farm workers		*	*			*
Crop handlers		*	*			*
Recreational users		*	*	*		*
Peripheral communities		*	*	*		*
Urban vegetable and fruit consumers, consumers inside and outside of the country		*	*			
Consumers of meat from cattle raised on pastures irrigated with wastewater					*	

to remain infectious after leaving its host. An intermediate host provides the conditions for an obligatory part of the pathogen life-cycle.

1. *Non-latent, low persistence*

This category includes viruses such as infectious hepatitis A, protozoa and some helminths. Transmission takes place via the faecal–oral route and is associated with personal hygiene and the domestic environment.

2. *Non-latent, moderate persistence*

This category includes bacteria such as those that cause shigellosis, typhoid and cholera that have extended survival periods in untreated wastewater.

3. *Latent, persistent, faecal–oral transmission without intermediate host*

This category includes *Ascaris* and some other intestinal helminths with a faecal-oral transmission route. Together with Category 4 it is considered the highest risk category in wastewater treatment and use. Eggs are likely to concentrate in sludge and some will remain in treated wastewater. *Ascaris* eggs may be found on harvested plants.

4. *Latent, persistent, soil-transmitted without intermediate host*

This category includes hookworms *(Ancylostoma* and *Necator* species) and some other intestinal helminths. They belong to the group of helminths posing the highest risk category in wastewater treatment and use. The eggs are likely to concentrate in sludge and some will remain in treated wastewater. The larvae hatch in moist soil and they infect the human host by penetrating the skin.

5. *Latent, persistent and with vertebrate intermediate host*

This category includes the bovine tapeworm and is important where cattle grazes on pasture irrigated with wastewater. People are infected when they eat insufficiently cooked meat. There is no equivalent parasite of sheep and goats.

6. *Latent, persistent and invertebrate intermediate host*

This category includes schistosomiasis, caused by trematode (blood fluke, genus *Schistosoma*) parasites, which spend part of their life-cycle in aquatic snails.

Assessing changes

At the core of the assessment process is the prediction of how the major health determinants are changed by the project and how these changes vary for each community group, each stage of the project and each locality. The assessment translates the relevant health hazards into health risk factors. The three principal risk factors are:

- community risk factors;
- environmental risk factors;
- institutional risk factors.

These risk factors are described with examples below. The consultants should establish how these will change, and the assessment will be halfway completed.

Community risk factors

There are many characteristics of a community that make it vulnerable to health risks. These include poverty, educational level, immune status, age, gender, training and place of origin. They can be subdivided into biological factors and lifestyle factors. For example, a poorly-trained and overworked workforce who must endure long night shifts for poor pay are vulnerable to occupational injuries.

In Africa, it is especially children and adolescents seeking refreshment in natural water bodies during the hottest time of the day who are most at risk of contracting schistosomiasis; the risk is exacerbated if they have not received hygiene education and if there is no access to adequate sanitary facilities in their community.

Wherever fetching domestic water from wells or other sources is the exclusive responsibility of women, there will be a gender-specific risk of skeletal and muscle injury.

Development will incur changes in the various hazards related to community risk factors; it may also introduce new hazards. As the composition of a community changes through resettlement, so will its immune status. Some community groups may benefit more from development than others, and as a result equity disparities within a community may increase.

Environmental risk factors

In an EHIA, both the physical and social environment require consideration. Projects often cause changes in both. For example, diverting, channeling and storing surface water can produce conditions in which malaria mosquitoes thrive. Resettling communities can produce insecurity and social disruption resulting in communal violence. Increased motorized transport is associated with an increased risk of injuries and accidents.

Examples of questions to consider include:
- Will there be adequate supplies of domestic water?
- What provision has been made for the safe handling and storage of hazardous chemicals?
- Have any measures been taken to improve traffic safety?
- Will the project affect the production of subsistence crops and are instruments in place to maintain the nutritional status of poor farming communities at an acceptable level?
- Could social disruption lead to an increase in the suicide rate?

Important lessons can be learned from studying the health impacts that resulted from similar projects that are already operational. The project design document and the preliminary outcomes of the feasibility study should shed light on the environmental and social changes that can be expected.

Institutional risk factors

Apart from the Ministry of Health, many governmental and nongovernmental institutions have responsibilities for protecting or promoting human health. The final component of the assessment concerns the capacity, capabilities and jurisdiction of health protection agencies. Together, these make up the institutional risk factors that may be changed by a project.

Capacity refers to the resources available in terms of staff, equipment and budget.

Capability refers to knowledge, skills and experience of staff to use the resources available optimally, and the framework that allows them to operate efficiently.

Jurisdiction refers to the power assigned to institutions to regulate or control certain aspects of a project.

An analysis of institutional risk factors will help identify gaps in institutional responsibility and accountability as well as the need to establish institutional arrangements that will support the intersectoral action needed for the proper implementation of the health management plan.

The section below presents an example of questions to ask concerning the institutional aspects of a proposed wastewater treatment plant, and why, in a real case scenario, a project failed to achieve adequate health protection.

Examples of questions to ask about a wastewater treatment project

- Who should determine whether the water quality output of the plant is acceptable?
- Should the Ministry of Irrigation make independent tests on the treated wastewater before accepting it?
- Who should determine what crops are grown in wastewater and how should this be monitored?
- Who should determine what method of irrigation is used and how will they decide if it is safe?
- Will the treatment plant be run at maximum safety at all times? What determines this?
- Which ministries/government officers should have access to copies of the WHO guidelines?
- What are the roles of the Ministry of Health and of the Environmental Protection Agency?
- How should a crop restriction or crop certification programme be administered?

Potential reasons for failure at a water treatment plant

WHO has produced guidelines for safe wastewater reuse, but in a recent health impact assessment it was found that these guidelines were not available to the project managers. Further investigation of the wastewater treatment plant suggested that it could fail for the following reasons, ranked in order of priority: poor management, lack of chlorine, excess influent of industrial waste, lack of electricity and equipment failure.

Staffing and management. The commissioning engineers were responsible for the sale and installation of the electro-mechanical equipment in the treatment plant as well as operation, maintenance and training for the first year. The handover period was likely to extend in practice from 1 year to 2–3 years, providing some opportunity to train local staff in correct operational procedures and hence increase reliability. However, the following management problems may have affected reliable operation of the treatment plant:

- managers below the Director occupied their positions reluctantly with little incentive or empowerment;
- there was little scope for reward for extra responsibilities, little accountability, little opportunity for staff development and no staff appraisal;
- salaries were very low.

Chlorination. The plant required some 600 tonnes of liquid chlorine per year. A one month supply was to be stored on site. It was unclear whether the transport and storage procedure was safe or whether any interruption in supply or dosage could be expected.

Industrial waste. It was unclear whether industrial waste could interfere with operation of the plant.

Power. The plant would generate 50%–90% of its own needs after the first six months and could cope with a loss of external power for up to 12 hours.

Equipment failure. The treatment plant was equipped with multiple standby equipment to reduce the likelihood of plant failure. It was designed to have an emergency bypass at both input and output, which diverts the flow down a covered culvert, to an open drain, that empties into a marshland.

Monitoring. The Water Pollution Control Unit at the Ministry of Irrigation was responsible for monitoring pollution of irrigation water. It was unclear whether the unit had plans to monitor the treated effluent and the resources to do so. The treatment plant would maintain its own laboratory for monitoring the quality of its product. It was unclear whether this laboratory had been designed to monitor helminth eggs or amoebic cysts.

Reaching a conclusion

When all the data have been gathered, analysed and cross-checked, it is necessary to reach a conclusion about the change in health risk for each health hazard identified. The data can usefully be summarized in a table (e.g. Table 2). For each health hazard the conclusion may be: increased risk, decreased risk or no change.

There are a number of health issues for which there are so many factors responsible that no simple conclusion can be reached. In these cases, it may be necessary to simply state the change in risk factors and consider whether any of the changes could be considered detrimental to human health in general.

Whatever the case may be, the purpose of the assessment is to formulate recommendations to safeguard human health, to mitigate health risks and to use opportunities for health promotion. This is the final stage of the assessment.

Table 2. Summary health impact assessment

Project title	
Location	
Exposed community	

Health hazards	Community risk factors	Environmental risk factors	Institutional risk factors	Change in health risks attributable to the project

Regularly, health impacts occur through complex sequences of events, which involve all three types of risk factor. In one north African country, for example, government policy promoted the settlement of nomadic tribes. As a result, the camel population dwindled and one particular type of vegetation, that camels used to feed on, expanded rapidly. This change in vegetation cover favoured the rodent population, which also expanded, and as a result an important outbreak of cutaneious leishmaniasis occurred. In this case, community risk factors changed, followed by environmental risk factors, and there was a gap in institutional responsibility to deal with the issue effectively.

Priorities

Faced with the wide range of health hazards associated with development, the planner must prioritize, regulate and monitor. Priorities should include hazards that are severe, affect large numbers of people or occur frequently. Regulations should include procedures for the implementation of health safeguards and mitigating measures by non-health sectors. Monitoring systems should be based on simple indicators that can be readily and cheaply measured and that change quickly enough for regulators to react. The quality of health sector data is rarely sufficient for indicator use as described here. It is most suitable for monitoring hazards with a low latency, such as communicable diseases, injuries and some forms of malnutrition. Complex biological or physical tests of low-level residues in high technology laboratories are expensive and cannot be reproduced on a wide enough scale. In countries of the Eastern Mediterranean Region, both of these problems are in evidence.

One method of prioritizing health issues in development is through proper economic evaluation, for example by considering costs versus benefits. Economic development is planned in order to promote growth and improve living standards. As such, its outcome is measured as a benefit–cost ratio. It should, however, also be planned to avoid increased health risks. Measuring the economic cost of ill-health is a more controversial issue. It can be measured in terms of lost production, lost school attendance, hospital treatment required, purchase of medicines, nursing care, pain and distress. It can represent a significant portion of the economic benefits of a development activity or it can even be higher than those benefits.

Over the past 15 years, the World Bank and the World Health Organization have made considerable progress in the development and use of a summary measurement of the burden of disease — the disability-adjusted life year (DALY), which considers the value of early death and disability [32]. Initially developed to support rational decision-making within the health sector, DALYs also have a potential to better anchor health in development negotiations and decision-making. At the time a Health Management Plan is negotiated (usually together with an Environmental Management Plan and a Social Action plan), it will need well-founded economic arguments. Both the costs of increased ill-health and the cost–effectiveness of proposed health safeguards and mitigating measures need to be covered.

The perception of health priorities is often driven by politics, fashion and fear rather than objective criteria. The major health hazards in the Region probably result from smoking practices, indoor air pollution, crowding, traffic injury and unhygienic food production, processing, preparation and storage, poor drinking-water quality and poor sanitation. The main health concerns of environmental agencies, however, are probably associated with residual pollution in air and water. These are concerns because of the fear that they may produce disease of high severity over a long period of time. Both kinds of hazard require regulation.

Regulation is available through two mechanisms. First, there is the environmental and health impact assessment framework for which environmental agencies are responsible. One of their duties is to regulate new large projects that may transform the physical environment. In order to manage their workload, they must move upstream to the regulation of planning policy. For example, the cumulative effect of many small processes may be more harmful to the environment and to human health than a small number of large processes. By addressing the issues upstream, at the policy level, important savings can be made in the impact assessment process.

Second, there is urban/town planning under the responsibility of municipal authorities. Such authorities are theoretically responsible for land planning and the supply of infrastructure. In setting the criteria for the development in these two areas health issues must be taken into consideration. In practice, however, rapid urbanization and the effects of the free market often overwhelm the municipal authorities. As a consequence, criteria are not strictly adhered to, suboptimal decisions are made and monitoring of impacts and compliance with regulations is inadequate.

Recommendations to safeguard human health/Health risk management

The final step in environmental health impact assessment is health risk management. It consists of incorporating health safeguards and health mitigation measures in project design, construction and operation. Safeguarding entails proposing modifications to project plans and operations and ensuring that the capability exists for effective mitigation. This could include strengthening of protection agency capabilities.

Mitigation entails vigilant monitoring for the lifetime of the project accompanied by appropriate and timely response to increasing health risks. Monitoring depends on an adequate health information system. Annex 2 provides an example on health mitigation measures in the Eastern Mediterranean Region. Possible mitigation measures could be grouped in to the following classes:

- opportunities for modifying project location;
- opportunities for modifying project design;
- opportunities for modifying project operation and maintenance;
- opportunities for incorporating environmental management measures;
- opportunities for strengthening health services;
- the need for monitoring and surveillance.

Each mitigation measure on the list should be classified in terms of affordability (Is it cheap to build?); sustainability (Is it cheap to maintain? Is it easy to operate?); acceptability (Is it socially acceptable to the local community?); accessibility (Is it physically, socially or economically accessible to the vulnerable communities?); and cost–effectiveness.

Examples

- In an agricultural project, one may choose to modify irrigation and drainage channel design and maintenance. The purpose is to improve water flow, prevent leakage and stagnation and prevent mosquito or snail breeding. The maintenance may be cheap if the community participates, but it may be difficult to motivate the community.
- In the context of most development projects, access to adequate sanitation can often be improved. The purpose is to ensure safe excreta disposal, prevent contamination of open water and prevent mosquito vector breeding and fly breeding. Social acceptability varies.
- Proper storage of chemicals and training of workers can help to prevent poisoning.

- Improved health centres can ensure that sick individuals receive adequate treatment. It may be difficult to recruit trained staff and to maintain drug supplies. Health centres can also be used for health education but this requires special skills and budgets and must be continuous.

All recommended actions should be compiled in a comprehensive and intersectoral health management plan. The latter includes all the health safeguards; health mitigating measures and health promotional measures and puts them in a logical framework with a clear indication of related budget and responsibilities. The health management plan also describes the arrangements and activities for effective monitoring during a project's construction and early operational phase. This involves the monitoring of community health indicators to ensure that when unexpected adverse health effects occur the health authorities can respond immediately. It also involves monitoring of the compliance by the project management with the agreed design and operational measures for the reduction of health risks.

The main point to remember about EHIA recommendations is to keep them practical. Suggest which agency would be responsible for the budget and which agency would be responsible for implementation. The best health safeguards are ones implemented by the

Table 3. Summary of recommendation features

	Recommendations
Project stage	
Timing	
Technical adequacy	
Specificity	
Social acceptability	
Cost	
Responsibility	
Capital or recurrent cost	
Fixed or variable cost	
Financial or economic cost	
Direct or indirect cost	

projects that do not require community behaviour adjustment. They separate the people from the project, or change the project design to achieve the same objective in a safer manner. Recommendations should be appraised for each of the main features stated in Table 3. The details of appraisal are presented in Chapter 5.

Chapter 5
Appraisal of EHIA studies

> This chapter covers the detailed actions required for quality assurance of the EHIA process, through independent appraisal. It proposes the components of a systematic approach to checking the methods and procedures used in the EHIA. As a first step, appraisal criteria need to be agreed and checked. Next, the chapter discusses ways by which the accuracy, comprehensiveness and sensitivity of the EHIA conclusions can be tested. Finally, it provides a framework for the appraisal of the recommendations that have emerged from an EHIA, with respect to their viability and to the soundness of their technical, social and economic aspects. This chapter draws importantly on the information provided in Health Opportunities in Development [33].

EHIA appraisal: purpose and functions

Appraisal is the quality assurance component in the EHIA procedure. Its purpose is to establish and maintain independent quality standards. This has immediate implications for the modalities and timing of the appraisal stage in an EHIA procedural framework. Appraisal is, in principle, a regulatory function for which the ultimate responsibility lies with government authorities. The group mandated to carry out the appraisal should be independent of the individual or group that was responsible for the actual EHIA. In practice, the final responsibility for the appraisal will be with the national EIA/EHIA Commissioning Authority. This arrangement facilitates the first step of any appraisal; to decide whether the EHIA conforms to the original terms of reference. Yet, it will also require that the National EIA/EHIA Commissioning Authority takes sufficient distance from the terms of reference it formulated itself and makes a frank evaluation of their adequacy. Retrospectively, it may find flaws in the terms of reference that may have contributed to the EHIA not meeting certain quality standards.

Reserving a time-slot for appraisal in the overall project cycle is essential. It must be carried out immediately after the submission of the EHIA report. Yet, there should also be enough time for an inadequate EHIA report to be sent back for further improvements and refinements, and for the formulation of a detailed health management plan that can be put on the agenda of the negotiations over project financing.

The national EIA/EHIA Commissioning Authority may require additional expertise to properly appraise an EHIA report. It is suggested that in contracting out the appraisal of specific technical areas, whenever possible, local expertise be used. Also, the independence of the exercise should be guaranteed through a legal requirement, such as the submission of a declaration of interest by each external partner that excludes the risk of political or commercial interests distorting the outcome.

Two stages can be distinguished in appraisal. First, the applied EHIA method and procedure and the basis for the final conclusions need to be verified. If this first stage identifies flaws in the EHIA, then these need to be corrected and the corrections need to be reflected in the recommendations, before the recommendations themselves can be appraised. The second stage, appraisal of the recommendations, should lead to the confirmation of elements to be included in the health management plan.

The outcome of any EHIA appraisal will be one of four possible positions of the national EIA/EHIA Commissioning Authority:

- the EHIA report is acceptable;
- there are minor flaws in the EHIA report that need revision;
- there are major flaws in the EHIA report that make it necessary to redo one or more substantive parts of the assessment entirely;
- the EHIA report is rejected as unacceptable.

Appraising EHIA method and procedure

The starting-point for any EHIA appraisal should be the terms of reference formulated by the National EIA/EHIA Commissioning Authority. An inventory should be made of the items in the terms of reference that are addressed in the EHIA and those that are not. In the light of new information that will have emerged, the adequacy of the original terms of reference should also be revisited, exonerating the consultants from any flaws that can be traced back to deficiencies in the instructions they received. Lessons learned from revisiting the EHIA terms of reference should be well documented for use in the formulation of future EHIA terms of reference for new projects.

Three important areas need in-depth consideration in the appraisal of the EHIA method and procedure:

- objectivity and bias, as functions of possible conflicts of interest, timing and availability of resources;
- the quality of the data gathering process, largely determined by the level of access to information;
- procedural rigour.

Objectivity is the first prerequisite of any acceptable EHIA report. It can be compromised by a number of issues: conflict of interest, timing, financial resources, access to information and procedural rigour.

Consultant's conflict of interest

There are a number of actors in the EHIA process whose interactions and mutual dependencies may create situations of conflict of interest that can affect the objectivity of the final report. In nationally supported projects, the EHIA consultant is likely to have been contracted directly by the project proponent. In projects that are externally supported, the consultant dealing with the health part of EHIA may be subcontracted by a larger consortium of consultants, dealing comprehensively with all preparatory studies required. In some instances, the EHIA consultant may be directly contracted by a bilateral or multilateral support agency.

Whatever the configuration may be, the customer relationship is likely to introduce some conflict of interest, which usually has to do with consultants trying to meet the expectations that are (or are thought to be) desirable to their patron. In this connection, an arrangement where an external donor supports the EHIA consultant directly is probably optimal.

The development of an organigram for the EHIA exercise, showing links and possible dependencies between the various actors will help identify any potential sources of conflict of interest.

Timing

There is an important difference between the time boundaries set for the EHIA through scoping, and the actual timing of the EHIA. Inadequate timing can greatly reduce the value of the EHIA report.

EHIA should be carried out and completed early enough to allow health impacts to become decision-making criteria in the consideration of different project options and, within a given selected option, the design alternatives. This is the most cost-effective way to ensure that a project meets its economic objectives as well as a number of sustainability objectives, including the protection and promotion of human health.

Even more upstream, a strategic impact assessment can consider health implications of new or adjusted policies. The level of sophistication of this approach does, however, limit its applicability.

If the assessment was carried out at the time when all key decisions for a project's implementation had already been taken, then the EHIA loses a considerable part of its value. Its recommendations will then be restricted to the operational phase.

The second issue related to timing concerns the opportunities of the health consultant to interact with consultants responsible for the feasibility study and the assessment of environmental impacts. Synergies and economies of scale in data gathering, and opportunities to analyse association between separate datasets will only be brought to realization if the timing of the assignments of the various consultants is properly synchronized.

Thirdly, the absolute amount of time spent by the health consultant is an indicator of the objectivity of the EHIA. Short assignments of a month or less will only allow for a desk study and meetings with key government officials. Arrangements of up to nine months will allow for broader consultations, including consultation of affected local communities, as well as a certain level of data collection through field surveys. In a time frame of several months there will also be real opportunities for coordination with those carrying out the feasibility studies and environmental assessment, and for iterative action resulting from such consultations. For some health issues, however, data collection over a full 12–month cycle may be necessary and this should also be taken into consideration in the appraisal.

Financial resources

The budget component allocated to EHIA may be the source of important biases in its conclusions. As a rough indicator, an adequate share for EHIA of the overall amount available for spending on the feasibility and design stages would be between 2% and 5%. In the more specific context of impact assessments, between 10% and 25% should have been allocated to the health component.

The appraisal should indicate an analysis of resources allocated and actually used for EHIA. Whenever this share is below the minimum indicated above, this is a signal to be aware of biases that may have resulted from excluding essential elements or cutting corners. An evaluation of the expenditures made on specific budget lines of the consultant (salary, subcontracting, travel, equipment and materials, etc.) will also reveal possible biases.

Access to information

There are many possible obstacles to obtaining all relevant information to arrive at balanced EHIA conclusions. One of the most important aspects of exploring the report's objectivity is to ensure it is sufficiently comprehensive and credible.

The EHIA consultant will have to collect a considerable amount of information from formal sources. The terms of reference should be accompanied by documents certifying the consultant's assignment and facilitating access to official documents. Nevertheless, key informants from different ministries may be reluctant to share information. The objectives of the EHIA may be perceived to be at odds with the sectoral interest of a ministry or authority, and those directly involved in the proposed project may fear undue delays resulting from the EHIA process. Research institutions may be selective as well in the information they provide, reflecting a bias related to their own areas of professional interest.

Different biases can come in when the consultant gathers data and information from local and affected communities. Such efforts may suffer from communication problems resulting from language barriers, or there may have been prejudices in contacts with local communities, related to race, gender or social structure. It is common that communities provide external consultants with information that reflects their expectations rather than reality.

Members of the national EIA/EHIA Commissioning Authority should first of all check the information sources quoted in the EHIA report against their own knowledge of available reports and documents. They should then investigate whether:

- existing reports were obtained from relevant ministries and authorities, and cited;
- information obtained from different sources was cross-checked;
- local consultants were employed;
- a wide range of key informants were interviewed;
- all sections of affected communities were considered and consulted.

Once the levels of comprehensiveness and credibility have been established of the information that forms the basis for the EHIA, the next step is to appraise procedural rigour.

Procedural rigour

Normally, the EHIA procedures described in Chapter 4 are followed by the consultant, yet it is the task of the appraisal team to establish whether they were applied with sufficient rigour. The various steps in the exercise must have been carried out with adequate breadth and depth, and with solid coherence between the steps.

The first question to ask is whether the consultant identified all important health hazards that could be associated with the project. In considering the individual health hazards identified, it is important to verify the datasets that led to their identification. They should be recent and reliable.

Next, the appraisal should ensure all vulnerable communities were included in the EHIA. The report should link identified hazards to vulnerable communities for the different stages of the project. Also, for each community it should describe in detail its various characteristics, and it should clarify how and to what extent changes in these characteristics, caused by the project, translate into health effects.

At the core of the appraisal is the detailed consideration of how the consultant has assessed the community, environmental and institutional risk factors as they result from project-induced changes in environmental and social health determinants. Checking procedural rigour involves finding answers to the following questions:

- Does the report identify how different community groups would be affected by the project?
- Does it identify the risk factors associated with each vulnerable community group?
- Does it describe the geographical distribution of health risks? In particular, does it discuss downwind and/or downstream effects?
- Does it identify potential zones of transmission or exposure?
- Does it give details of seasonal distribution of health risks?
- Does it distinguish risk factors in construction, early operation (first 5 years) and late operation (5–20 years)?
- Does it identify all institutions relevant to health?
- Does it identify their strengths and weaknesses?
- Does it identify the health services strengthening needs that could arise from the project?

The appraisal report should cover these issues *in extenso*, and summarize in detail any deficiencies or mistakes encountered. It should also consider how the findings for individual hazards have been synthesized into a final, overall assessment. In particular, the arguments supporting the synthesis, and the weighting of various components into one integrated assessment need to be scrutinized.

Appraising the conclusions

Synthesis of all the different findings makes up the next step towards the formulation of conclusions and ranking them by priority. These include the findings with respect to the affected communities and identified community groups, with respect to the range of health hazards and how their risk levels change as the project gets underway, and the specific risks linked to specific project stages.

For example, construction workers moving into a malarious project zone will run a high risk of becoming infected if they themselves come from non-malarious areas. The risks will be reduced by the promotion of coping behaviour (use of insecticide-treated mosquito nets, wearing protective clothing at peak mosquito biting hours, compliance with the prescribed use of prophylactic drugs) and by improving the quality of the temporary housing facilities. If a large part of the construction team falls ill, this will have important consequences for the project's timely completion. If, in the early operational phase of a project, resettled families move in, also from non-malarious areas, the hazard may continue to be the same (unless major environmental management measures to reduce mosquito breeding have been deployed as part of the project). Yet, the community group at highest risk will be young children, and the use of insecticide-treated nets will be more prominent among preventive measures. Non-immune adults may also fall ill in a sequence of outbreaks, and the economic output of the project may be severely undermined. Yet, the time horizon (years rather than months for the construction workers) will cause a shift in the economic evaluation of safeguards and mitigating measures as well, and a change in the emphasis within a range of interventions, from more capital-intensive infrastructure to more service-oriented recurrent ones.

Another example, this one illustrating the different risk levels for a diversity of community groups at the operational stage, is the increased use of pesticides that tends to accompany irrigation development. The hazard of exposure to pesticides and their residues has several pathways with implications for different groups in a community. The first and most obvious group are the farmers applying the pesticide in the field. Without proper training and protective clothing and devices, their risks are significantly increased with the intensified use of these chemicals. Depending on the prevailing methods of collecting and using domestic water, the exposure of community members in general may also increase, particularly where water is collected from drainage canals or from shallow wells. Pesticide residues may percolate into shallow groundwater and contaminate the wells. Pesticide storage will need to meet certain standards to keep the toxic products away from children, and to also discourage their use for suicide. Incorrect application of pesticides may create food safety hazards within the community or for outside consumers. In countries where the presence of pesticides and their residues in food is strictly regulated, incorrect applications may undermine the economic basis of a community and ultimately result in poverty and malnutrition.

Accuracy

The quality of the evidence base for the conclusions is of critical importance. If the information on which the conclusions are based is not accurate, the resulting recommendations will lack credibility. Not only can this be checked by referring back to the original sources of information, but a cross-check with information in the other impact assessment (environment, social) and feasibility study reports may also help identify discrepancies.

In direct surveys and studies carried out for the assessments, accuracy can be undermined by faulty sampling procedures, sample sizes that are too small, or inadequate statistical analysis. It is recommended to always ensure the services of a reputed statistician at this stage of the appraisal.

Comprehensiveness

In combining the datasets of the various assessments of different hazards at different project stages, the comprehensiveness of the overall exercise may suffer. It may also have proved impossible to gather equally reliable data from all areas covered by the originally established EHIA scope, and this may distort the comprehensiveness of the final conclusions.

Sensitivity

The assumptions made during the entire EHIA process will play an important role in determining the level of probability of the conclusions. The terms of reference should have instructed the consultants to diligently document in the report the assumptions they made. It is therefore important to test individual assumptions for their sensitivity, by applying the extreme values of a probable range and observe what effect this has on the conclusions of the assessment. If the conclusions are not significantly affected by this analysis, then they can be considered robust.

Completion of the appraisal of the EHIA conclusions signals a critical decision-making moment: if the EHIA methods, procedures and conclusions are deemed acceptable, then the second part of the exercise can be undertaken. If, however, important flaws have come to light in the EHIA report thus far, then these will have to be addressed before the proposed recommendations can be appraised.

Appraising the recommendations

EHIA recommendations consist of health safeguards, mitigating measures and health promotional measures. Their implementation can be part of the project design, or it can take place during the construction and/or operational phases. The responsibility for carrying out recommended measures may lie with different sectors, but usually the project proponent and the health authorities play key roles. The health authorities have the mandate to verify and certify compliance with all health-related measures during all phases of a project.

In traditional EIAs, the consideration of health aspects would invariably lead to recommendations aimed at strengthening the health services to address health problems resulting from, or exacerbated by, a development project. This "after-the-fact repair" approach [8] put the responsibility for health exclusively with the health sector and ignored the important role other sectors can play in maintaining or improving the health status of affected communities. The economic, sustainability and environmental aspects of taking health into consideration as a cross-cutting issue and at an early stage of any development were entirely overlooked.

A properly carried out EHIA provides the basis for specific recommendations responding to identified health risks for a given community group and at a given stage of the project. Recommended measures either divert risks entirely, minimise adverse health effects or add value to a project by exploiting health opportunities.

Recommended measures can be of different types, including regulatory measures, technical design and operational changes, economic tools (subsidies, taxes, incentives), and strengthening of health services.

The recommendations contained in the EHIA report can be appraised for three distinct criteria: technical adequacy, social acceptability and economic feasibility. It is recommended to systematically appraise all recommendations by listing them in a table with a column for each of these three criteria.

Technical adequacy

The technical adequacy of recommended measures is linked to issues of project design, the implications for project operation and maintenance, opportunities and restrictions imposed by the geophysical setting and the local climate, and the local availability of materials.

In many instances, the design, operation and maintenance aspects in a given setting are straightforward. Examples of functional solutions with no other implications include the incorporation of a double spillway in the design of a dam in areas where there is a risk of blackfly breeding (vectors of onchocerciasis), or the incorporation of self-draining hydraulic structures in irrigation schemes where schistosomiasis is a problem. The often advocated cement lining of irrigation canals to prevent seepage and the formation of pools where malaria vectors can breed is, however, already less self-evident. Canal lining requires considerable initial investment, and there are a range of different lining materials, each with its own advantages and disadvantages. Cement lining will initially prevent seepage, but in the longer term cracks will lead to more seepage at specific points in the irrigation scheme. This measure would only be technically justified if (1) it has additional benefits, such as saving scarce irrigation water and (2) it can realistically be expected that a canal maintenance plan can be implemented during the entire life of the project.

For many recommended measures, the design, operation and maintenance issues may become irrelevant in specific geophysical or climatic settings. Clearly, where remote communities are affected by a project, it is not realistic to rely on regular access by the health services to address the associated health problems. Relatively expensive project design interventions may be the only technically viable solution. The often quoted example of the impossibility of having farmers in hot climates using boots to protect them from schistosomiasis infection in irrigation schemes is, in part, another illustration of technical inadequacy; it also relates, however, to the criterion of social acceptability.

Social acceptability

The technical adequacy of recommended measures may be excellent, yet they become irrelevant if they are not accepted socially. There may be specific sociocultural characteristics that play a role in acceptability levels in affected communities, and these may be well known beforehand. It should not be forgotten, however, that these characteristics themselves may change as a result of the project, and that acceptability patterns and levels will change with them.

Growing urban populations throughout the Eastern Mediterranean Region will shift their traditional nutritional patterns, with direct consequences for their health. At the same time, growing demands for certain products will change agricultural production patterns, often causing change in environmental determinants of rural health. Government policies on food security, including food subsidies, will further modulate the picture and will call for strategic impact assessments, in addition to more conventional project-wise EHIAs.

Mechanisation of agriculture is often rapidly accepted by communities: farmers can clearly see the advantages of a mechanised approach to agricultural production. It may be as difficult to promote health safeguards in the context of a development that is otherwise very readily accepted by communities, as it is to promote measures that come up to barriers of social acceptability. Yet, an impact assessment will often point out the risks of increased accidents and injuries as a result of mechanisation.

An overall increase in socioeconomic status may render time-tested interventions useless, because communities perceive them as backward and unsophisticated compared to the measures their newly-gained wealth provides them access to.

Incorporation in the EHIA report of the outcome of a study of the knowledge, attitudes, practices and beliefs of vulnerable communities is a good indicator of whether or not the consultant has taken social acceptability aspects into consideration in the formulation of recommendations. The illiteracy rate is an important consideration when recommending measures that involve written instructions, such as labels on pesticides. Attitudes towards sexuality may determine the success rate of condom promotion in the fight against HIV/AIDS. Certain traditional practices, particularly among tribal groups, may have unknown health dimensions. And religious convictions may hamper the impact of health safeguards.

Finally, an adequate level of public hearing as part of the assessment process will also provide certain guarantees that the measures recommended meet with social acceptability requirements. It is even better if a participatory approach has been applied to the actual design of the measures, and the assistance of a cultural anthropologist can facilitate this. Depending on their technical sophistication, the measures themselves can also rely on a certain level of community participation.

Economic feasibility

It should never be forgotten that, in the final negotiations on the elements of the health management plan, economic arguments will outweigh all other types of arguments. Therefore, not only should the EHIA terms of reference indicate that recommended measures should be supported by an economic evaluation of possible alternatives, but a considerable part of the appraisal should be spent on checking the economic evaluations done. In brief, appraisal of the economic aspects of the recommended measures will ensure that:

- the cost estimate of recommended measures is complete;
- the recommended measures are affordable;
- the most cost-effective option has been chosen and there are no hidden costs;
- the costs of recommended measures are significantly offset by the costs that would be incurred to the health sector in the absence of any measures.

Of the various methods of economic evaluation (cost–effectiveness analysis, cost–benefit analysis, cost–utility analysis), cost–effectiveness analysis is generally accepted to be the most appropriate. This holds especially true since the introduction of the burden of disease concept, which provides a generic effectiveness indicator, the disability-adjusted life year (DALY), a summary measure of community health.

The first question to address is whether the EHIA report includes an economic evaluation of the recommended measures. Such an evaluation should include a cost estimation and an effectiveness measurement. The comprehensiveness of the financial analysis of the cost should be complimented by considerations relating to economic values, and should bring in capital costs, recurrent costs, opportunity costs and the discount rate. The affordability of recommended measures will, to a large extent, depend on their direct costs in the context of the national budget, external support in the form of loans and grants, the national foreign debt and related debt payments, and the implications for operation and maintenance costs in the long term.

In the end, the Ministry of Finance will not only want to know whether recommended measures are affordable, but also whether they represent value for money, in other words, are they the best measures limited resources can buy?

Placing the costs of recommended measures in a broader context is also important. Sometimes engineering interventions as health safeguards may turn out disproportionately expensive when compared to the health services expenditures required if no measures are taken at all. There have also been examples where certain project elements were disguised as health measures in order to boost the project's internal rate of return.

It is strongly recommended that the services of a health economist be obtained to advise the appraisal team on these issues.

At the end of the appraisal exercise, a report is written with all findings, and with the final verdict concerning acceptance or rejection of the EHIA. It is important not to let the perfect overshadow the good. The perfect EHIA report does not exist, and with recommended measures addressing major health issues, the impacts will be dealt with to the extent possible. The measures should be developed into a solid health management plan with a realistic budget that can be submitted and defended at the subsequent negotiating sessions with the Ministry of Finance.

References

1. *Health impact assessment: harmonization, mainstreaming and capacity-building. Report of a WHO interregional meeting* (Arusha, 31 October–3 November 2000). Geneva, World Health Organization, 2001 (WHO/SDE/WSH/01.07).

2. WHO European Centre for Health Policy. *Health Impact Assessment, Main Concepts and Suggested Approach.* Gothenburg Consensus Paper. Copenhagen, Denmark, WHO Regional Office for Europe, 1999.

3. *Human health and dams. The World Health Organization's submission to the World Commission on Dams.* Geneva, World Health Organization, 2000 (WHO/SDE/WSH/00.01).

4. UNDP. Human development report 2003. *Millennium development goals: a compact among nations to end human poverty.* UK, Oxford University Press for the United Nations Development Programme, 2003.

5. Cooper-Weil DE, Alibusan AP, Wilson JF, Reich MR & Bradley DJ. *The impact of development policies on health. A review of the literature.* Geneva, World Health Organization, 1990.

6. *Our planet, our health. Report of the WHO Commission on Health and Environment.* Geneva, World Health Organization, 1992.

7. *Health and environment in sustainable development – five years after the Earth Summit.* Geneva, World Health Organization, 1997.

8. WCED. *Our common future, Report of the World Commission on Environment and Development.* Oxford, Oxford University Press, 1987.

9. United Nations Conference on Environment and Development – UNCED. *Agenda 21, Programme of Action for Sustainable Development.* New York, United Nations, 1992.

10. *Alma–Ata Declaration and Health for All Strategy.* Geneva, World Health Organization, 1978.

11. *World Health Assembly Resolution 35.17 Health implications of development schemes.* Thirty–fifth World Health Assembly Geneva, 3–14 May 1982 (http://policy.who.int/cgi-bin/om_isapi.dll?infobase=WHA&softpage=Browse_Frame_Pg42. html, accessed 21 January 2005).

12. *World Health Assembly Resolution 45.24 Health and development.* Forty–fifth World Health Assembly Geneva, 4–14 May 1992 (http://policy.who.int/cgi-bin/om_isapi.

dll?infobase=WHA&softpage=Browse_Frame_Pg42. html, accessed 21 January 2005).

13. Ghebreyesus TA et al. Incidence of malaria among children living near dams in northern Ethiopia: community-based incidence survey. *British Medical Journal,* 1999, 319:663–666.

14. Tiffen M. *Guidelines for the incorporation of health safeguards into irrigation projects through intersectoral cooperation.* PEEM Guidelines Series 1. Geneva, World Health Organization, 1991 (WHO/CWS/91.2).

15. WCD. *Dams and Development. A new framework for decision-making. Report of the World Commission on Dams.* London, Earthscan, 2000.

16. Birley MH. *Guidelines for forecasting the vector-borne diseases implications of water resources development.* PEEM Guidelines series 2. Geneva, World Health Organization, 1991 (WHO/CWS/91.3).

17. Birley MH, Gomes M, and Davy A. *Health aspects of environmental assessment.* World Bank, Update 18 to the Environmental Impact Assessment Resource Book. Washington DC, An Update of the World Bank Environmental Sourcebook, 1997.

18. *The world health report 2003. Shaping the future.* Geneva, World Health Organization, 2003.

19. Jobin W. *Dams and disease, ecological design and health impacts of large dams, canals, and irrigation systems.* London, E and FN Spon, 1999.

20. Mara D, and Cairncross S. *Guidelines for the safe use of wastewater and excreta in agriculture and aquaculture.* Geneva, World Health Organization, 1989.

21. *Health guidelines for the use of wastewater in agriculture and aquaculture. Report of a WHO scientific group.* Geneva, World Health Organization, 1989 (WHO Technical Report Series 778).

22. Bos R. Boundaries, health impact assessment and integrated vector management. In: Casman EA, & Dowlatabadi H, eds. *The contextual determinants of malaria.* Washington DC, Resources for the Future, 2002.

23. Birley MH. *The health impact assessment of development projects.* London, HMSO, 1995.

24. Health Canada. *A Canadian handbook on health impact assessment.* Ottawa, Ministry of Public Works and Government Services, 1999.

25. Birley MH, and Peralta G. *Guidelines for the health impact assessment of development projects.* ADB Environment Paper 11. Manila, Asian Development Bank, 1992.

26. Ewan C, Young A, Bryant E, Calvert D. *National framework for health impact assessment in environmental impact assessment.* Australia, University of Wollongong, 1992.
27. Ministry of Health. *A guide to health impact assessment. Guidelines for public health services.* Wellington, New Zealand, 1995.
28. Department of Health. *Philippine national framework and guidelines for environmental health impact assessment.* Manila, Philippine Environmental Health Services, 1997.
29. Overseas Development Administration (ODA). *Manual of environmental appraisal. Revised edition.* London, Overseas Development Administration, 1992.
30. Dahlgren G, Nordgren P, Whitehead, M, eds. *Health impact assessment of the EU Common Agricultural Policy.* Stockholm, Swedish National Institute of Public Health, 1996.
31. *Human health and climate change: risks and responses.* Geneva, World Health Organization, 2003.
32. The World Development Report 1993. *Investing in health.* Washington DC, World Bank, 1993.
33. Bos R, Birley MH, Furu P, and Engel CH. *Health opportunities in development. A course manual on developing intersectoral decision-making skills in support of Health Impact Assessment.* Geneva, World Health Organization (in collaboration with the Liverpool School of Tropical Medicine, the Danish Bilharziasis Laboratory and the Institute of Education of the University of London), 2003.

Annex 1
Examples of environmental health problems from the Region

Introduction

In this annex examples are presented from seven representative areas in the Eastern Mediterranean Region with regard to environmental health problems, the main hazards of relevance, communities at risk and possible mitigating measures. It also documents mitigating measures that have been taken by government agencies. It evaluates the suitability and effectiveness of these measures from a public health point of view.

The annex provides arguments in support of EHIA through concrete examples, and it serves as an "information source" to refer to for background on typical environmental health problems associated with development projects; the underlying hazards and particularly vulnerable communities.

The situation with regard to health, environment and development linkages is described for seven areas selected to illustrate both common features and the diversity of the Region. The selected areas reflect a variety of situations with regard to human settlements (i.e. the urban/rural mix); population density; natural resources; environmental conditions; types of development activities (policies, programmes and projects); and institutional and administrative structures and arrangements.

The seven areas are referred to as Areas I to VII (see Tables A1 to A5). Names of countries are not given since the areas were selected to represent eco-epidemiological situations. Readers of this guide working in the Region will find information in this annex that is relevant in part or as a whole to their local situation, irrespective of the administrative or political framework within which they are working.

The aim of this annex is to review linkages between environmental problems in the Region and their associated health hazards and risks. A health hazard refers to a potential to cause ill-health. A health risk indicates the level of probability that the potential is realized.

The environmental problems discussed in this annex follow the categories identified by the majority of governmental authorities responsible for the environment and/or for environmental health. These categories are:

- water pollution;
- air pollution;
- soil pollution;
- pollution by solid wastes;
- informal settlement areas.

Not all the desired information was readily available at the time data were collected. Where complete datasets were available, as was the case for water pollution, environmental problems and their associated health hazards and risks were identified for each of the seven areas. Otherwise, as in the case of informal settlement areas, only some of the areas are reported upon, or else a general note has been made. All information in this annex comes from official sources, such as government reports.

Types of environmental problems and their health impact
Water pollution
Area I

Water pollution in this area is considered a serious environmental problem because the water basin is a closed one. As a result, all pollutants entering the basin will end up in surface water (one of the rivers), or in groundwater (wells and springs). Thus, two categories of water pollution in this basin can be identified: surface water pollution and groundwater pollution.

Pollution of surface water and main health hazards and risks

The two main sources of pollution in the main river of the river system, which crosses the urban as well as the rural part of Area I, are domestic and industrial wastewater, which are estimated to cause 60% and 40% of the river's pollution, respectively.

Domestic wastewater originates from the large population of the main city and its periurban area, estimated to be 3 million in total. The severity of pollution from domestic wastewater can be explained by the fact that the ratio of domestic wastewater to natural water in the main river and its tributaries is 1.38 to 1.

Industrial wastewater comes from 250 factories and 170 tanneries. Almost all of these industries release their effluents without any treatment.

The main sources of pollution of the other (minor) rivers in the system are considered to be domestic wastewater and agricultural run-off, containing pesticide and fertilizer residues.

Coliform analysis of surface water in Area I suggests that it is highly contaminated by sewage. Most coliform counts are in the range 1000–100 000/100 ml. The pollution problem intensifies in the dry season when the flow in the rivers decreases.

Chlorinated pesticides, some of which are banned (DDT, and its metabolite DDE), have been detected in surface waters, especially those downstream of one of the main agricultural areas. Nitrogen levels were high, especially downstream of the main city. The concentration of nitrogen in the lower portions of the main river reached 25–70 mg NO_3/L. This suggests a significant sewage and industrial wastewater discharge into the river system.

Heavy metal pollution was also identified as a serious problem in surface water. Very high levels of chromium (40 mg/L) were detected in surface water near the industrial area where the tanneries are situated. The chromium was detected in its reduced form, which is less toxic to humans. However, an oxidation process by chlorination, for example, can change it to its hexavalent form which is extremely toxic to humans. Heavy metal pollution of surface water is likely to be a serious problem in many industrial areas of Area 1.

Among the important health risks associated with the hazards resulting from surface water pollution feature:

- communicable diseases, such as parasitic infections, hepatitis A, summer diarrhoea and typhoid;
- noncommunicable diseases, such as heavy metal toxicity.

Health risks can increase when untreated surface water is used for irrigation or when the pollution reaches the groundwater that serves as a source for the drinking-water supply. Agricultural land which extends from the rural to the periurban part of Area I is already irrigated with wastewater. Health risks from contaminated surface water have not been evaluated in any detail in official reports. A Ministry of Health report shows, however, that 70% of the population in the agricultural production zones of Area I is infected with intestinal parasites. It has been suggested that the main reason for this high prevalence is the use of wastewater for irrigation.

Pollution of groundwater and the main health hazards and risks

There are 23 500 wells in the main (rural/periurban) agricultural part of Area I. These are used as a source of potable water for rural communities. They are also used for irrigation and industry.

The main sources of groundwater pollution in the Area are industrial and domestic wastewater and agricultural wastes. Types of pollutants identified are chemical and bacteriological. The former is indicated to be serious. High levels of two banned chlorinated pesticides (dieldrin and heptachlor) were detected in groundwater in a subdistrict of the area. The levels of these two pesticides exceeded the national drinking-water standards (0.03 micrograms per litre).

Nitrate concentrations in another sub-area in the main city were almost as high as the upper limit of the WHO drinking-water standard (50 mg NO_3/L) or even higher. The sources of nitrates are the seepage of untreated sewage and excess fertilizers.

Fortunately, heavy metal pollution can not be considered a problem in groundwater in this area. All groundwater samples met the national drinking-water standard for heavy metals.

Health hazards and exposure pathways are similar to those mentioned above. Waterborne disease accounts for 18.2% of all diseases in this basin. This is made up of typhoid (2.5%), cholera (0.2%) and other waterborne diseases (15.5%).

Corrective measures for Area I may include: disinfection of rural wells, control of excessive use of agricultural pesticides, and treatment of tanneries effluent, at least through chemical precipitation of chromium.

Area II

Pollution of the main river and its lake and the main health risks

The main sources of pollution to the river and its lake are the following.

- Industrial activities: Many large and small industries are established along the river. These industries dispose their untreated effluents directly into water courses. The main water polluting industries are:
  - the fertilizer industry in the main city which is a source of nitrates;
  - tanneries in the second city which are a source of chromium;
  - soap industries in both cities which produce effluents rich in alkaline substances, oxidants and organic matter.
- Domestic sewage.
- Hospital wastes – there are 64 hospitals in the Area.
- Agricultural activities.

One of the main health hazards identified in official reports is the high level of nitrates deposited in the river and its lake. The main health risks associated with drinking-water polluted with high levels of nitrate are blue-baby syndrome and long-term carcinogenic impacts.

The high concentration of nutrients present in the lake is the main reason for the important growth of blue algae, especially at the end of the summer season, indicating severe nitrate and phosphate pollution.

Because of the high level of pollution of the lake, its water is no longer used as a source of potable water for the two main cities of Area II. This reduces the potential health risk of using such polluted water, but at the same time deprives the populations of these two growing cities of an ample water supply.

Pollution of groundwater

The main sources of groundwater pollution are agricultural activities and domestic sewage. The principal health risks are communicable diseases, such as typhoid, summer diarrhoea and parasitic infections; and noncommunicable diseases which may arise from the high levels of nitrates, phosphates or pesticides in the groundwater. Again, this risk increases when polluted water becomes a source for domestic use. The probability of health risks occurring as a result of this type of pollution is high because of the geological characteristics of Area II which allows pollutants to enter into the aquifer.

The communities at risk are the inhabitants of the villages in the mountainous part of Area II since their wells suffer from domestic sewage pollution. Other communities at risk are the inhabitants of the adjacent plain and its town. It is worth noting that the wells used as a source of potable water for the town are polluted by agricultural wastes. The level of this pollution has not been measured however, making it difficult to estimate relevant health risks.

Area III

This represents a coastal zone with major petrochemical industries.

Pollution of coastal waters

The main sources of water pollution in this basin are:

- untreated domestic waste resulting from sewerage outlets which pass the effluent directly into the sea. Moreover, in winter, floods carry wastes from the sewerage outlets into the sea resulting in severe pollution episodes along the coast;
- untreated sewage from tourist complexes;
- untreated industrial wastes;
- hospital wastes;
- oil pollution from oil refineries and oil barrages;
- use of some prohibited fishing methods (i.e. the use of chemicals to kill fish).

There is also pollution resulting from external sources located outside the national water boundaries. The impact of this type of pollution is considered considerable since the sea in question, the Mediterranean, is semi-closed with highly-populated coasts. Some 200 000 industrial establishments are located on the Mediterranean coast, about 90% of them on the European coastline. Moreover, pollutants carried by some major European rivers end up in this sea. Pollution along some parts of the Eastern Mediterranean coastline is exacerbated by the fact that self-purification needs relatively extended periods of time due to high levels of salinity.

The main health risks which have their origin in pollution of coastal waters in Area III are:

- communicable diseases, such as cholera and dermatological and fungal diseases;
- noncommunicable diseases, such as chronic or acute chemical poisoning.

These health hazards can result from eating contaminated sea food or from swimming in the coastal waters (direct contact with various types of pollutants). More research is needed to identify the communities at risk, from among both local residents and tourists, and estimate health risks more accurately.

Pollution of ground and surface water

The level of pollution of potable water supplies is considered serious according to official reports. The sources of this type of pollution are considered to be the following.

- Expansion in sanitation and sewerage networks in the towns and villages of the area. The outlets of these networks are usually located in valleys near residential areas. The wastewater is usually not treated and is increasingly posing a threat to potable water supplies. Arbitrary construction of sewage bore-holes also contributes to the contamination of nearby artesian wells used for irrigation and drinking purposes. This type of pollution is considered serious, especially since the geological characteristics of the area allow pollutants to percolate quickly into the aquifer.
- Increased use of hormones and pesticides in livestock and agricultural production, especially on the coastal plain where many greenhouses are established. This may lead to pollution of potable water supplies through agricultural run-off and contamination from livestock excreta.

The main health risks which may result from pollution of potable water supplies in the coastal area are communicable diseases, such as typhoid, summer diarrhoea, hepatitis A and amoebic dysentery. Noncommunicable diseases may also result from pollution of potable water supplies, including carcinogenic effects caused by long-term exposure to chemicals and hormones. More research is needed in order to specify and better estimate health risks posed by such pollution, including geological, hydrological and epidemiological studies.

Area IV

Water pollution in this basin has not been discussed explicitly in official reports. However, the severity of water pollution especially in Area IV's main river has been indicated in several official sources. The main sources of water pollution are:

- industrial effluents – the main water-polluting industries are battery-producing industries, tanneries, metal-plating industries and soap and oil extraction industries;
- agricultural run-off which usually contains pesticide and fertilizer residues;
- untreated domestic sewage.

The main health risks resulting from water pollution in the basin occur when contaminated water is used for irrigation or drinking purposes. High levels of arsenic were detected in vegetables grown in contaminated soils and irrigated from the polluted river.

Area V

The main sources of water pollution in Area V are:

- untreated domestic wastes from urban and rural centres;
- industrial wastes;
- agricultural wastes.

Water pollution is not considered serious in Area V because of the high rate of flow of the river which can reduce pollution levels.

Area VI

Pollution of groundwater, especially of wells, is considered to be serious. The main source of pollution is agricultural production (fertilizer and pesticide residues). The principal health hazard consists in the high level of nitrates in some wells used as a source of potable water. The main health risk of nitrates in potable water occurs after its conversion to nitrites in the human digestive system. Nitrites have the potential to cause blue-baby syndrome, especially in bottle-fed infants.

It can be concluded that the communities at risk are those using these wells as a source of their potable water. The seriousness of the problem can be inferred from the fact that 20 wells in Area VI have been closed. However, the location of the polluted wells has not been exactly identified in the official reports.

Area VII

Until recently water pollution was not identified as an environmental health problem in this basin. However, water pollution is increasing as a result of population increase and the continuous expansion of agricultural activities, especially irrigation schemes.

High levels of salinity and fluoride are detected in well-water. This makes it an unsuitable source of potable water. Local environment authorities identified no water pollution problems in this basin. Local health authorities stated, however, that "... some wells in the area contain a high level of fluoride that represent a risk to the health of the users of these waters".

Air pollution

Area I

Air pollution is considered a major environmental problem in the capital city. The main causes of air pollution are:

- transport, which is responsible for 70%–80% of air pollution;
- industries such as tanneries, cement factories, glass and fabric industries;
- crafts which use primitive methods of production and which are located in residential areas, mainly in informal housing areas;
- domestic heating during the winter season, especially the traditional heating devices which can cause indoor air pollution.

The health risks vary according to the type of pollutant, its concentration in the air and the mode, time and frequency of exposure. Respiratory diseases, eczema, ophthalmic diseases and cancers are all examples of health hazards which result from different types of air pollution. The incidence of these diseases occurring in polluted environments is 3–4 times higher than in non-polluted ones.

The communities at risk are those living in areas with high pollution levels, inhabitants of informal residential areas and those whose occupational activities result in high exposure levels to air pollutants, such as transport workers and traffic police. Especially vulnerable community groups are children, elderly people and those suffering from respiratory, allergic or cardiac conditions.

Area II

Official reports show air pollution to be an environmental problem in the major city. The fertilizer industry and the oil refinery are identified as main sources of air pollution. Figures in official reports show that the level of certain air pollutants, such as ammonia, nitrogen oxide and sulfur dioxide, exceed the WHO standards by many times. The poisonous gas hydrogen sulfide, H_2S, has been also detected in the air – government regulations prohibit any traces of this gas in the air.

The main health risks are airborne diseases, such as acute respiratory diseases (e.g. allergic reactions), chronic respiratory conditions (e.g. emphysema which results from long-term exposure to air pollutants), ophthalmic diseases and carcinogenic effects.

One study gave evidence of the high percentage of cancers in Area II relative to other parts of the country. The study concluded that "the incidence of cancers is the highest in the country. The number of new cases reported annually represents a quarter of all cancer cases reported in the country". The study recommended that Area II's main city should be treated as an industrially polluted city from the environmental and epidemiological point of view. The study, however, did not establish a clear link between industrial pollutants and the various types of cancer which occurred in the city. The study may have neglected the impact of tobacco smoking.

Area III

Many large industrial plants, especially public sector plants, are located along the coastline and near or inside large residential areas. Air pollution is considered an environmental problem in one of the main towns and its surrounding villages and in the main port and its neighbouring areas. The main sources of air pollution in the former are an oil refinery and its power station. A cement factory and the loading of phosphate in the port are considered to be the main sources in the latter. Moreover, exhausts from vehicles contribute to air pollution.

The main health risks are related to respiratory diseases. The risk level associated depends on the weather conditions, the type of air pollutant, its concentration in the inhaled air and the time of exposure to specific pollutants. Vulnerable community groups are the same as those referred to under Area I above.

Statistics in 1992 show that 34% of patients who visited health centres in Area III had respiratory problems. Data on patients visiting three health centres in distinct locations during the first eight months of 1994 show that:

- 76% of the patients who visited a health centre adjacent to the cement factory were diagnosed as suffering from respiratory problems;
- 50.7% of patients who visited a health centre whose catchment area includes people living near the power plant and oil refinery were reported to be suffering from respiratory diseases;
- only 14% of patients who visited a third health centre, located away from main pollution sources, were reported to have respiratory diseases.

Area IV

Air pollution is considered a main environmental problem in Area IV's main city, characterized by a dense cloud of smoke and dust hanging over the city centre. The main sources of air pollution are battery-producing factories, transportation and cottage industries located in residential areas.

Official reports mention high levels of lead in many of the residential areas of the city. A ban on leaded gasoline would lead to a rapid reduction of this particular hazard. The main health hazards are airborne diseases.

Soil pollution

Official reports identify soil pollution in agricultural land as one of the main environmental problems in many countries. Soil pollution can be hazardous to health if plants intended for human consumption are grown in contaminated soils or when soil pollutants, such as fertilizers, pesticides and heavy metals percolate to groundwater which is used for irrigation and drinking purposes. Health risks from soil pollution depend on the type of pollutants, their concentrations in the soil and their biodegradability.

There is little or no information on measurements of soil pollution in many of the countries. This makes it rather difficult to assess the health risks resulting from it. General examples of soil pollution, its causes and its main health hazards are drawn from Areas I, II and IV. Besides its impact on food safety, the main impact of soil pollution is chemical pollution of groundwater.

Area I

The main sources of soil pollution in this basin are:

- industrial effluents especially from lead smelting and lead–liquid battery-producing factories;
- uncontrolled use of pesticides and fertilizers especially the use of illegal pesticides and the use of fertilizers containing hazardous material;
- contamination by solid and hazardous wastes.

Contamination by heavy metals such as lead has been reported. For example, high levels of heavy metals were detected in parsley grown in the area.

As explained above, health hazards and risks can vary according to a multitude of factors.

Area II

The main sources of soil pollution in this basin are:

- industrial effluents mainly from the phosphate fertilizer industries and the wool industry;
- agricultural wastes, especially contamination by pesticides and fertilizers;
- pollution by solid and hazardous wastes.

Health risks which result from soil pollution in this basin can turn more severe when soil pollutants percolate to shallow aquifers used as a source of drinking-water. This is more likely to occur in many areas in this basin because of the local geological characteristics.

Area IV

The main sources of soil pollution in this basin are indicated to be the same as those encountered in Area I. The most serious health risks result from consuming vegetables grown in soils contaminated with high levels of heavy metals. Analysis conducted on vegetables grown for human consumption in soils contaminated by heavy metals and irrigated from Area IV's polluted river water showed high levels of arsenic – three times higher than the level allowed for humans and animals.

Pollution by solid waste

Solid waste is made up of domestic, hospital and industrial components. These can be considered as a serious environmental problem and pose several health hazards because of the following factors.

- *The mode of disposal of solid wastes.* Most solid waste is disposed of in landfills, many of which are located on the outskirts of cities and are considered illegal. Untreated solid waste is also disposed of in exposed rubbish tips outside cities and towns. These exposed waste disposal areas have the potential to cause serious health risks, such as infant diarrhoea and dysentery, because they provide conditions conducive to the propagation of flies and rats. Moreover, highly toxic substances can be present in hospital and industrial wastes. Hospital waste represents a health hazard because it may contain, among others, toxic chemicals and contaminated syringes with related serious health risks, such as HIV or hepatitis B infection.
- *The low efficiency of plants treating solid wastes.* Generally only few waste treatment plants are available. Most of these plants are old and do not have the capacity to treat the large quantities of waste of major cities.
- *Scavengers or waste pickers.* Scavengers search the rubbish tips for disposed cans, plastic containers, bones, bread and food leftovers. Many of the waste pickers are children. Health risks to those waste pickers may include hand and leg injuries, intestinal and respiratory infections, eye infections and exposure to hazardous waste. Additionally, some of the recycling processes can be hazardous. The reuse of collected bread and food as an input in human food, of collected plastic containers for preserving food and drinks and of polluted egg cartons to hold sweets and food all imply serious health hazards to the consumer.

Rapid urbanization and informal settlement areas

Many cities are growing quickly because of increased migration from rural areas, but also because of high internal demographic reproduction rates; rapid and uncontrolled urbanization is the result. Increasingly, this phenomenon is putting pressure on the limited infrastructure and services in urban centres. Many of the migrants have settled in informal settlements inside or around cities. These informal residential areas have grown rapidly and are now home to a substantial proportion of the population of cities. For instance, and this is not an extreme example, in one of the Region's capital cities, an estimated 406 900 people (27% of the city population) live in 14 informal areas.

Illegal residential areas are usually highly populated and overcrowded. The housing in these areas lacks basic health standards. The air quality is poor, both indoors and outdoors. Proper systems for sewerage and for the distribution of potable water are absent. The residents in these informal areas obtain their potable water supplies from any of the following sources:

- an illegal distribution network connected to the water source of formal residential areas;
- illegal wells which are not inspected;
- other water sources located near to the residential area, such as lakes, rivers and springs;
- purchased water. This water is usually expensive and frequently not safe.

Other basic services, such as health centres, are also absent in these areas. This combination of poor living conditions and lack of basic services and public health infrastructure can, according to the findings of official reports, lead to the outbreak of diseases, such as acute respiratory infections, tuberculosis, pneumonia, influenza, meningitis and intestinal infections. Unconfirmed reports indicate that waterborne diseases, such as cholera, typhoid and diarrhoea, exist predominately in informal settlement areas.

Contamination from sewage is another major problem. This is because sewage flows in shallow open drains which are very close to water supply sources and illegal connections running along the surface of the ground. Injuries are common in these areas. These usually result from illegal electrical networks and dangerous and illegal energy supply connections.

A concrete example of the health situation in the informal residential sector comes from an investigation reported in a government study of an informal residential area in a periurban zone. The population in this area is estimated to be around 250 000. No legal potable water supplies are available in this area nor is any kind of sewerage system. Wells used as a potable water supply in the area are all polluted. Additionally, wells which were dug 10 km away from the area also showed the same level of pollution. Statistics conducted by the health centres serving this area showed a high level of diarrhoea and typhoid, especially among children under ten years old.

Table A1. Area I environmental problems, causes and examples of associated health impacts

Environmental conditions	Health hazards	Causes and examples of health impacts
Water pollution	• Untreated domestic wastewater • Untreated industrial effluents • Agricultural wastes	Communicable diseases: e.g. 70% of the population in one a sub-area have parasite infections. Noncommunicable diseases: heavy metal toxicity and carcinogenic effects (e.g. chromium salts from tanneries or chlorinated chromium salts), agro-chemical poisoning which may result from chloro-organic compounds in potable well-water.
Air pollution in urban centres Outdoor: Indoor:	• Transport (70%–80% of air pollution in the main city) • Industries, e.g. crafts and small industries (usually in informal residential areas) • Domestic heating in winter • Overcrowded accommodation in informal areas	Noncommunicable diseases: Many air pollutants, e.g. nitrogen oxides (No_x), sulfur dioxide (SO_2), carbon monoxide, total suspended particulates (TSPs), are usually 3–4 times higher than WHO standards in many locations in the main city. Exposure to these pollutants causes respiratory diseases, eye diseases and fatigue. Heavy metal poisoning, for example from lead.
Soil pollution	• Industrial effluents • Fertilizer and pesticide residues • Solid wastes	Pollutants containing hazardous ingredients and heavy metals are the main cause. Health risks to consumers of vegetables grown in contaminated soils or to those who use water which has percolated through contaminated soil. High levels of cadmium, lead, chromium and arsenic were detected in parsley grown in polluted soil in one sub-area.
Pollution by solid wastes	• Illegal landfills and exposed rubbish tips • Low efficiency of plants treating domestic wastes • Absence of incinerators in hospitals	Health risks are: • Intestinal infection, such as infantile diarrhoea and dysentery, which can affect communities exposed to rubbish tips (e.g. waste collectors, consumers using polluted recycled waste materials as food containers). • Infections resulting from contact with hospital wastes contaminated with HIV or hepatitis viruses or with industrial wastes containing toxic chemicals. • Hand or leg injuries to waste collectors.
Informal residential areas	• Rapid urbanization • Growing migration from rural areas to the main city	A lack of healthy conditions, sanitation, potable water supplies and health services and the presence of illegal polluting crafts result in several health risks e.g. meningitis, acute respiratory infections, pneumonia. Noncommunicable diseases include injuries such as electrical shocks.

Table A2. Area II environmental problems, causes and examples of associated health impacts

Environmental conditions	Health hazards	Causes and examples of health impacts
Water pollution	• Domestic sewage • Agricultural activities • Industrial activities • Hospital wastes	Pollution, by nitrates, pesticide residues, of wells used for potable water in one town. The health risks associated with this type of pollution are agro-chemical poisoning, blue-baby syndrome and long-term carcinogenic impacts. Domestic sewage pollution in wells used as a source of potable water in the mountain areas, in the plain and in the town. The main health hazards are communicable diseases, such as typhoid, parasite infections and poisoning by chloro-organic compounds.
Air pollution	• Industrial activities especially in and around the main city • Transport	Air pollutants, e.g. NO_x, SO_2, TSPs, are present in high concentrations at certain locations in the city. H_2S, a poisonous gas, is also detected in the air. The main health hazards are airborne diseases, such as respiratory diseases, asthma and eye diseases. Cancers are identified to have a high incidence in the city (a quarter of all cancer cases in country).
Soil pollution	• Phosphate fertilizer effluents in the main city and wool industries in the second city • Agricultural wastes, such as pesticide residues • Solid wastes	Local geological characteristics allow soil pollutants to enter into the aquifer used for irrigation or drinking purposes. The level of contamination of groundwater is far more serious than that encountered in surface water. The main health hazards are noncommunicable diseases, such as phosphate poisoning or heavy metal poisoning.
Pollution by solid wastes	• Illegal landfills and exposed rubbish tips • Low efficiency of the waste treatment plant in the second city	Health risks are: • Intestinal infection, such as infant diarrhoea and dysentery, which can affect communities exposed to rubbish tips (e.g. waste collectors, consumers using polluted recycled waste materials as food containers). • Infections resulting from contact with hospital wastes contaminated with HIV or hepatitis viruses or with industrial wastes containing toxic chemicals. • Hand or leg injuries to waste collectors.
Rapid urbanization and informal residential areas	• Growing migration from rural areas to cities	Informal residential areas were not officially identified as a problem in the Area. However, these are likely to be present in a rapidly growing city such as the main city. Health hazards to residents would be the same as those identified in Table A1, i.e. A lack of healthy conditions, sanitation, potable water supplies and health services and the presence of illegal polluting crafts result in several health risks e.g. meningitis, acute respiratory infections, pneumonia. Noncommunicable diseases include injuries such as electric shocks.

Table A3. Area III (Coastal zone) environmental problems, causes and associated health impacts

Environmental conditions	Health hazards	Causes and examples of health impacts
Water pollution	• Untreated domestic sewage • Untreated industrial wastes • Agricultural run-off • Oil pollution • Use of prohibited fishing methods	Communicable diseases, such as dermatological infections resulting from swimming in polluted waters. Communicable diseases resulting from contaminated groundwater are typhoid, summer diarrhoea and parasitic infections. Noncommunicable diseases resulting from contaminated sea or groundwater are: chemical poisoning by pesticides or fertilizer residues (acute and chronic); heavy metal or chemical poisoning resulting from consuming contaminated sea food.
Air pollution	• Industrial emissions from oil refinery and power station, from cement factory and from phosphate loading in port town • Vehicle exhausts	Certain air pollutants (SO_2, NO_x) exceed by many times the WHO thresholds. H_2S is also detected in some villages around refinery town. Dust is found in high concentrations around port town. The main health hazards are respiratory diseases and eye diseases. Of patients who visited a health centre adjacent to the cement factory, 76% had respiratory infections.
Pollution by solid wastes	• Illegal landfills and exposed rubbish tips especially on the coast • Unsuitable bore-holes • Low efficiency of waste treatment plant	Communicable diseases, such as typhoid and summer diarrhoea which result from leaching of pathogens into groundwater used for irrigation and drinking purposes. Injuries to individuals who scavenge from these landfills.
Informal residential areas	• Random distribution of residential areas in the countryside and on fringe of cities or along the coasts	A lack of healthy conditions, sanitation, potable water supplies and health services and the presence of illegal polluting crafts result in several health risks e.g. meningitis, acute respiratory infections, pneumonia. Noncommunicable diseases include injuries such as electric shocks.

Table A4. Area IV environmental problems, causes and examples of associated health impacts

Environmental conditions	Main factors	Causes and examples of health impacts
Water pollution	• Industrial effluents • Agricultural run-off • Domestic wastewater	Main health hazards are: • Noncommunicable diseases, such as heavy metal poisoning, agro-chemical poisoning (acute and chronic). • Communicable diseases such as parasitic infections, typhoid and other viral infections. These health hazards result from using polluted waters for irrigation or drinking purposes.
Air pollution	• Industrial emissions in the main city, especially those from battery factories, cement industry, incinerators and quarries • Vehicles using lead-containing gasoline	High levels of lead are present. The main health hazard resulting from exposure to lead is fatigue, headache and neurological effects. High levels of dust are present especially in areas around quarries and incinerators. The main health hazards are respiratory diseases and eye diseases.
Soil pollution	• Industrial effluents such as those from lead smelting and liquid battery factories • Use of illegal pesticides on agricultural land • Use of fertilizers containing hazardous material	Main health hazards stem from heavy metal pollution. Vegetables grown in polluted soils in agricultural land contain high levels of arsenic (three times higher than the threshold).
Pollution by solid wastes	• Illegal landfills and exposed rubbish tips • Low efficiency of waste treatment plants • Untreated hospital wastes (72 hospitals)	Health hazards are the same as those mentioned in Table A1 under pollution by solid wastes.
Illegal residential areas	• Increased immigration	A lack of healthy conditions, sanitation, potable water supplies and health services and the presence of illegal polluting crafts result in several health risks e.g. meningitis, acute respiratory infections, pneumonia. Noncommunicable diseases include injuries such as electric shocks.

Table A5. Area V, VI and VII environmental problems, causes and associated health impacts

Environmental conditions	Health hazards	Causes and examples of health impacts
Area V		
Water pollution	• Agricultural wastes (fertilizers and pesticides)	Pollution of groundwater by nitrates is serious. In the main town, 20 wells have been closed. The health hazards are blue-baby syndrome and carcinogenic impacts in the long term.
Information is not available about other environmental conditions. This makes it difficult to assess health risks.		
Area VI		
Water pollution	• Agricultural wastes • Untreated domestic wastes • Industrial wastes	Not serious because of the high rate of flow of the river.
Area VII		
Water pollution	• Salination	High levels of fluoride are present in wells used for drinking. The main health hazard is fluorosis.

Measures to mitigate environmental problems and their health implications

Generically, there are several categories of measures that can be deployed in response to the problems observed in the above tables. They include:

- treatment of sewage and of industrial wastewaters, including nitrogen removal through extensive aeration;
- microbiological surveillance of sea food if any marketed, and surveillance of heavy metals content in the flesh of fish;
- physicochemical treatment of offensive industrial effluents;
- industrial exhaust-gas cleaning through dust removal and acidity neutralization.
- the establishment of controlled sanitary landfill, far from city limits, to be outside of the walking range of scavengers.

Measures for control of water pollution

An example of a specific measure undertaken or proposed to control water pollution in countries of the Region is the establishment of monitoring points along river systems in order to measure pollution levels. Samples are taken for the analysis of chemical (including heavy metals), and microbiological (including coliforms) contents. Monitoring results are, in some cases, circulated to all polluting industries and to the water users. Water quality is also monitored at certain points along the coast in order to assure its suitability for swimming.

Following are examples of institutions responsible for monitoring water pollution:

- Directorate of Potable Water of the Ministry of Housing and Utilities, responsible for monitoring potable water quality. This Directorate may also be responsible for monitoring effluents from wastewater treatment plants.
- City Water Supply and Sewerage Authority, responsible for testing water quality at the municipal level.
- Directorate for Public Water Pollution Prevention, usually part of the Ministry of Irrigation. The Directorate is responsible for monitoring industrial effluents and for directing the owners of establishments which are violating pollution standards to comply with proper corrective procedures. The Directorate is supposed, usually, to report any establishment that fails to comply with the responsible minister if it is in the public sector or to the governor if it is in the private sector.
- The General Directorate of Ports, responsible for monitoring pollution in national coastal waters.
- The Water Authority, responsible for monitoring water and wastewater quality.
- The Ministry of Health responsible for drinking-water surveillance.

Presently, few or no reports on the effectiveness of monitoring procedures exist. It may be assumed, however, that monitoring water quality is weak because of the technical limitations of the monitoring authorities. For example, in one country, the national water quality testing laboratory can analyse only 30 samples a day for general water quality analyses. The laboratory is not equipped to adequately detect pesticides and their residues, disinfection by-products or pathogens. Moreover, its instruments are old and unreliable, and neither repair services nor replacement parts are available. To protect public health the capacity of monitoring authorities need urgent strengthening. The equipment used for monitoring water quality should be upgraded to provide reliable and frequent tests for toxic chemicals, heavy metals and pathogens, especially in potable water.

It is also important to identify clearly the institutions responsible for monitoring and enforcement of standards and the arrangements to deal effectively with violations are discovered. An evaluation of the regional and national coordination between various agencies responsible for monitoring water quality will be useful in this context. Key functions and measures include:

- Standard setting for the quality of industrial and commercial wastewater which is allowed to be disposed into the sewerage system. In some cases, the institution responsible for setting the standards has not been identified and formally charged with the task by the country's authorities. Additionally, no clarification has been made of the nature of these standards (i.e. national or international standards).
- Sewerage systems and a wastewater treatment plant have been developed in most major cities. Many other urban settlements and the majority of rural areas, however, have no such service.
- Reuse of reclaimed wastewater in irrigation is proposed or already undertaken in some countries.
- Establishment of treatment plants for industrial waste, such as tannery effluents, has been proposed or undertaken.
- Some industries have started to establish their own treatment plants, for example, government-owned tanneries in one country, fertilizer industries in another and an oil refinery in a third country. It is not clear, however, whether all relevant industries are obliged to have their own treatment plant or whether they are establishing them on their own initiative. Institutional responsibilities for enforcement also require further clarification.
- In some countries, an anti-pollution control zone has been established around certain water resources, such as lakes and springs.

Measures undertaken to mitigate air pollution in urban centres

- In most cases, monitoring air pollutants in cities, where it occurs, is undertaken by specialized centres that are located in and mainly serve the capital city. Most such centres have only recently been established. There is not yet sufficient monitoring capacity to meet national needs.
- An example of a successful intervention comes from a major port city where the method of loading phosphate into cargo ships was changed to cause less pollution. This has resulted in reduction of pollution levels in the neighbouring areas. There is no indication, however, whether or not the air quality has evolved satisfactorily.

Other proposed measures to mitigate air pollution are:

- improving the quality of petrol and diesel fuels, and particularly reducing the diesel fuel's sulfur content;

- reducing the lead content in petrol;
- checking vehicles annually and setting standards for their exhausts;
- locating polluting industries away from cities;
- maintaining combustion devices in the established industries and removing particulate and other polluting gases from their exhausts;
- developing less polluting domestic heating devices;
- introducing regulations to prevent pollution and incorporating environmental considerations when constructing or modifying industrial establishments and when planning new towns;
- withdrawing licenses which permit the use of old polluting vehicles, to be completed in phases over a number of years.

Measures to mitigate pollution resulting from solid wastes

- Plastic containers made from reused plastic residues are prohibited as containers for food. This measure is to be implemented through cooperation between industrial, inspection and health agencies. Efforts should include raising public awareness.
- Raising farmers' awareness of the need not to use untreated wastewater.
- The Ministry of the Environment, in a number of countries, has formed a committee to inspect violations by hospitals and health centres regarding their methods of waste disposal.
- Increase and up-grade factories for regenerating solid wastes, including providing incinerators to cater for hospital wastes.
- Improve solid waste management through expansion of waste collection services. Provision of waste containers and transport facilities. Increasing the frequency of waste removal in some crowded areas.

Measures proposed to control informal residential areas

- Identifying existing areas of informal settlement and preventing the expansion or the establishment of new ones.
- Providing these areas with basic infrastructure and services, such as potable water networks, sewerage systems, electricity and health and education services.
- Preventing the establishment of any industry which is not suitable from an environmental point of view in informal residential areas.

Annex 2

A critical review of EIA/EHIA in the Region, with particular reference to development activities in the private sector

Background

In many countries in the Eastern Mediterranean Region, the procedure for granting environmental permits, including EIA, is the only formal procedure that gives consideration to the health impacts of development projects. The rationale of the exercise reported here is to reconsider the EIA process with a view to strengthening its health component, and thus to contribute to capacity-building for EHIA.

In most countries of the Region, the responsibility for environmental permits for development projects falls under one or more of the following: local authorities, the environment protection agency and the Ministry of Health. The procedure for granting environmental permits is, in most cases, the only formal procedure that gives consideration to the health impacts of development projects.

The national economy in many of the countries is government dominated. The private sector is, however, gradually playing a greater role, including taking over several public sector functions. In many countries of the Region new laws and regulations have been enacted, in recent years, mainly to encourage privatization and private investment. Generally, there are three types of enterprise: public, private and joint public/private. Major industries are still owned by the state, but several privately-owned industries have emerged, most of them concentrated around the main urban centres.

The data processed and reported in this annex came from EIA work done between 1994 and 1996 in selected representative countries of the Region. During this period, over 90% of applications (741 applications from the private sector) for environmental permits resulted in the conditional granting of a permit. However, it must be noted that most of the industries and projects subjected to EIA screening were small-scale ones, i.e. "assumed" to only have limited environmental/health impacts. In addition, most of them were already established so that the focus of this review is retrospective rather than prospective. It is also interesting to note that despite the fact that protection of human health was a primary concern in EIA and was always included in the required mitigation measures, little was achieved in practice.

Approach used in compiling and analysing data

The data were obtained from official sources in selected representative countries. The raw data included applications for environmental permits and the EIA responses to them for the period 1994–96. In many instances, the applications were already roughly categorized according to the year and the industrial sector. The proposed mitigation measures were attached to the government EIA responsible agency.

The following criteria was used to process the data:

1. *The sector.* These were mostly industrial or service sectors.
2. *The project.* These included textile, paper, plastic, food, metal and chemical industries and quarries.
3. *Project ownership.* Private, public or joint public/private ownership. However, most were private.
4. The name of the project (e.g. metal plating or clothes design).
5. The name of the project owner.
6. Location of the project.
7. Proposed mitigation measures:
   - mitigation measures proposed as conditions for all environmental permits granted by the EIA authority;
   - mitigation measures related to the project's physical establishment;
   - mitigation measures related to the project's inputs and outputs;
   - mitigation measures related to the production process;
   - mitigation measures related to workers and the workplace.
8. The date of submission of the application and the date of the response from the EIA authority.
9. The response from the EIA authority was as follows:
   - a permanent environmental permit;
   - a temporary environmental permit (i.e. concerned industry should relocate within a certain period (maximum of five years) to an industrial zone);
   - an objection to granting the environmental permit.

   Analysis of the health component was carried out by classifying mitigation measures related to health into three broad categories:
   - occupational safety and health;
   - consumer safety and health;
   - environmental health.

It is proposed that the procedure followed and the outcome of the review of environmental applications and permits should form the basis for establishing an EIA/EHIA database.

Comments on the findings of the critical review
Shortcomings in health-related mitigation measures

Most of the proposed environmental, as well as health mitigation, measures were general ones. Health mitigation measures typically include conditions such as provision of sanitary facilities, waste removal and ensuring application of occupational health and safety regulations.

From the review the following points need to be highlighted.

1. Mitigation measures were established only to prevent health risks occurring under normal working conditions. No account was taken of health risks which might occur due to accidents, such as spillages or explosions. Though the probability of accidents occurring might be low in many cases, the health risks encountered as a result of an accident might be very high.
2. Proposed mitigation measures concerning consumer health were very general. For example, the mitigation measure which required complying with the conditions established by the Ministry of Health when packaging a product, did not identify what these conditions were.
3. Mitigation measures concerning the use of control measures in the workplace lacked comprehensiveness and specificity. The references to requirements imposed by the Ministry of Labour and Social Welfare did not indicate what those requirements were. In the chemical industries proposed control measures included only those relating to individual workers, for example the use of protective gloves and masks. Even in this case control measures for specific production processes were not specified. Moreover, no mention was made of other engineering control measures, such as local exhaust ventilation. This was the case even for the metal and chemical industries which result in hazardous airborne pollutants, such as metal dusts, solvents and other toxic fumes and vapours. It should be noted that personal protective equipment is the worker's last line of protection from health hazards encountered at work. This type of equipment may actually cause health risks if it is not used and maintained properly.
4. There was no mention of how mitigation measures, including those related to health, would be enforced or what institution(s) were responsible for monitoring compliance. If monitoring is not rigorous enough, industries (especially those posing a greater health risk) would not implement the mitigation measures proposed by the environment/EIA authority.

5. No monitoring and inspection procedures were specified for small factories where the probability of health risks to workers or neighbouring communities is higher than in large industries.
6. No specification was made regarding hygienic conditions required during the production process. This is especially important in the food industry where a failure to comply with such hygienic conditions could result in considerable health risks to consumers.
7. Children are more vulnerable to occupational diseases than adults. However, in the best of cases, only in two industries (paper and metal industries) was the condition of "preventing the work of children under 16" mentioned. Gender-related vulnerability seemed largely to be ignored. The same is true with regard to health of "peripheral communities", i.e. communities at the periphery of the project.
8. Very few or no government projects were reported to be assessed despite the fact that in many countries they constitute the majority of development projects. Also, there was little or no reference to tanneries which is an industry with relatively high health risks.

Difficulties encountered by institutions granting permits

The main difficulties encountered by the environment/EIA authorities granting environmental permits were as follows.

Limited capacity

Capacity of these institutions is limited due to limited numbers of staff and limitations in their technical capabilities. In one country, where development activities were of a significant scale, there were only six staff, including the Director. This is a very low number in view of the huge volume of work that the staff have to cope with. Moreover, the technical capabilities of the staff should be strengthened, especially with regard to EIA/EHIA methods and related tools.

Lack of enforcement and legislation

The absence of a legislation which identifies institutional responsibilities in relation to environmental protection is a major obstacle. Environmental Protection Acts and EIA decrees are mostly in draft. Where this is the case, there is no legal basis for enforcing them. The environment/EIA authority has no legal power to enforce or monitor the implementation of its permit conditions and requirements. Its advice is carried out optionally and when considered as convenient by other government agencies such as local authorities. Health legislation often provides a well-established and strong basis for legal action on environmental health issues. Food safety and occupational health are a case in point. Such legislation could, with little modification, effectively be used in the EIA context. The legal perspective provides a strong argument in favor of the establishment of a strategic alliance between environment and health authorities.

Limitations of cooperation and coordination with relevant agencies

In many cases, the environment/EIA authority seems to have formal or informal cooperation and coordination links with other relevant government agencies which are not used effectively. However, this may partially due to the fact that the environmental laws are not yet enacted. As such, the environment/EIA authority does not yet have the power of a law enforcement agency. Consequently, its status and to some extent its appeal and negotiating powers, with other agencies is limited, especially when conflicts of interest arise.

Other issues

Response time

In most cases the response time to environmental permit application was one to three weeks, when perhaps one to three months would seem more appropriate for a thorough examination. Only on a very few occasions was the one to three week response time exceeded. This could be seen as a very good record, given the fact that one of the main objections to EIA is that it could delay project implementation and consequently economic development. It must, however, be noted that the limitation of resources of the environment/EIA authority constrains EIA activities. That is to say, the good response time pointed out here is not entirely due to competence, but is partly influenced by the limits of what can be done.

Economic costs

It was not possible within the scope of this work to evaluate the economic costs. It is essential that this is done, since it represents another objection to conducting EIA/EHIA of development projects.

The issues of relevant institutional framework, capability and capacity, administrative organization and intersectoral cooperation are discussed below.

Conclusion and recommendations to improve health considerations in proposed mitigation measures

The results demonstrated that the work of EIA authorities mainly covers small-scale private projects in the industrial sector located in or around the capital city. Several types of development projects were not covered. These include road construction, road transport industries, wastewater reuse, waste disposal sites, ports and harbours. As far as health is concerned, EIA authorities primarily consider a limited and out-of-date list of environmental and occupational health risks largely biased towards noncommunicable diseases.

Many countries depend heavily on water resources development projects. These are primarily agricultural schemes located all over the country, but mostly in rural areas. A considerable proportion of these schemes, especially of the larger-scale ones, are within the public sector. Communicable diseases, injury, nutritional conditions and psycho-social disorders need to be given sufficient consideration to balance the current bias towards noncommunicable diseases.

Health mitigation measures should be the result of a health impact assessment conducted on the project in question

This is recommended since it was observed that in many instances EIA committees were setting the same mitigation measures for different industries posing varying health risks. Small projects with no potential major health risks may conduct rapid health impact assessment using related guidelines. However, more detailed health impact studies may sometimes be necessary for projects with a high potential for health risk. Additionally, the health risks of process malfunction and accidents should always be considered and relevant preventive and mitigation measures proposed. An inspection system should be entrusted to check if mitigation measures are actually enforced and if they are working as proposed in the assessment.

Improve infrastructure and institutional capacity

It is recommended that all facilities required for inspection should be provided. For example, transport means are required for the EIA/EHIA committees undertaking inspection. Other basic facilities such as office space and computers should be provided.

In order to improve institutional capacity, training courses for the staff of the central EIA authority should be provided. These courses should generally provide the staff of the EIA/EHIA authority with a better understanding of broad health issues associated with development projects, and in particular occupational health and safety, and environmental health issues.

Training is needed to enable staff to carry out various levels of EHIA, from screening through initial examination to full EHIA. Both health and non-health personnel, can be trained to undertake the preliminary phases of EHIA.

Establishing and strengthening EHIA management information systems is an urgent need. Ministries of Health need to review and strengthen management information systems including aspects, such as coverage, data recording, transmission, compilation, analysis, reporting, timeliness, feedback and use by senior and middle level managers and by other health workers.

Research capacity needs to be built up by health professionals and institutions. Collaborative research with established regional and international centres would be appropriate in this regard.

A good research capacity is important for sustaining EHIA activities. Equally important is access to adequate and good quality health and environment information.

Ensure high-level support for EHIA

In some cases, current health policies and legislation and goodwill may be sufficient for conducting a successful EHIA study. In other cases, a fresh policy statement committing the country to EHIA would facilitate carrying out relevant activities. Ideally, a clear policy statement backed with appropriate legislation should be a near future goal.

Strengthen institutional cooperation and coordination

This is required in order to improve the quality and prospects of implementation of health and safety component in proposed mitigation measures. In addition to the already mentioned strategic alliance between health and environment ministries, cooperation and coordination should be strengthened between the Ministry of Health and the Ministry of Labour and Social Affairs, as well as with all other institutions responsible for enforcement and monitoring, such as local authorities. Improved intersectoral cooperation with the Ministry of Health and the Ministry of Labour and Social Affairs will involve health and safety specialists (which the environment authorities usually lack) in the EIA/EHIA committees.

Intersectoral collaboration is a prerequisite for a successful EHIA of development projects. Multisectoral effort involving the health, environment, development planning and implementation sectors are essential in this regard.

A number of intersectoral collaboration mechanisms already exist in many countries. For example, at the higher level of government there are usually a Higher Planning Council and a Higher Council for Environmental Safety, both usually headed by the head of government with all ministers acting as members. The Higher Planning Council is responsible for the development planning cycle, usually a five-year cycle. The EIA authority, the Ministry of Health, the Ministry of Labour and Social Affairs and other relevant governmental agencies have the opportunity through this Council to appraise and comment on all planned projects. They could therefore enhance EHIA activities through this important Council and improve them, while at the same time increasing their commitment and capacity and improve their capabilities and those of other relevant sectors in this regard.

There are usually intersectoral collaboration mechanisms at the technical and middle-management level, such as an Intersectoral Health and Environment Committee (ISHE) with representation from the Environment Department, the Ministry of Health and other relevant sectors. However, in many cases the Ministry of Labour and Social Affairs is not a member of such a committee. Inviting the Ministry of Labour and Social Affairs should be considered to ensure inclusion of occupational health and work–environment issues. Most of these committees are relatively new and not fully active. However, most seem to have taken or are proposing EHIA as their major focus.

An ISHE committee is a very good complement, with regard to EHIA intersectoral collaboration mechanisms, to the Planning and Environmental Safety Councils. The latter usually operates at the "higher" policy and programming level, conducting its work at infrequent intervals, while the former is a standing body that deals with current and on-going activities and can deal, hands-on, with any development project as it comes up for approval at the implementation level.

The ISHE committee can be a very good intersectoral collaboration mechanism if its membership, leadership, administrative setting and mandate are inclusive and appropriate. Also, such a committee would bring together EHIA and EIA.

The following suggestions should be considered in the formation of an ISHE committee and the establishment of its function:

The ISHE committee brief and activities with regard to EHIA need to be worked out in detail from the outset. The committee needs to be strong at the leadership level and at the coordinator level so that it becomes fully functional and effective. The leader should be a senior staff member of the Ministry of Health at the level of Director General or Deputy Minister. This will help elevate the committee status in front of its members from other sectors and give its activities, comments and decisions due weight. Perhaps equally if not more important is the need to select a coordinator for the committee from the health sector. The coordinator should be strongly interested in the subject. He/she should have a clear appreciation of the concept, necessary approach and of the relevant issues. More importantly he/she should have excellent communication skills and be able to relate easily to professionals from other backgrounds/disciplines/sectors. He/she should be aware of the multidisciplinary and multisectoral dimension of the subject and be clearly fit to coordinate such a committee.

A key duty of the ISHE committee will be to review and comment on EHIA study reports, prepared by consultants for major development projects.

As for the health sector, a working group should be formed to take responsibility for EHIA and related activities. This should be high-powered with a chairperson at the deputy minister level. The coordinator post should be jointly held by the head of occupational health and the head of environmental health units. Additionally, statistics and research and epidemiological surveillance units need to be represented. Also the academic medical institutions, for example the Department of Community Medicine/Faculty of Medicine, and the medical unit of the Social Insurance Department of the MOLSA should be represented as subsectors within the larger health sector. The former is important for providing academic/research input to the committee, while the latter would reflect labour ·health issues. Health impact of development on the workers is a substantial and integral component of EHIA. The workforce represents a significant vulnerable community group in all types of projects.

Define institutional responsibilities

Responsibilities of institutions undertaking monitoring and enforcement for EIA/EHIA should be defined clearly. This should be done in order to increase the efficiency of the monitoring procedure.

Glossary

Definitions of terms important in the context of environmental health impact assessment are presented in alphabetical order. Related terminology is clustered under the first entry.

Appraisal A critical examination of an identification report, which selects and ranks the various findings and solutions from points of relevance, technical, financial and institutional feasibility, and socioeconomic profitability, and precedes the approval by the authorities of the proposed action.

Also:

Assessment An examination in order to decide (as opposed to **analysis** an examination in order to understand).

Evaluation As systematic and objective an examination as possible of an on-going or completed project or programme, its design, implementation and results, with the aim of determining its efficiency, effectiveness, impact, sustainability and relevance of its objective, with the purpose of guiding decision-makers on future projects.

Agro-chemicals Chemical used in agriculture, such as fertilizer, pesticides and herbicides. Also referred to as chemical inputs.

Burden of disease A measurement of the gap between the current health of a population and an ideal situation in which everyone in the population reaches old age in full health.

Disability-adjusted life year (DALY) A summary measure of population health. One DALY represents one lost year of healthy life and is used to estimate the gap between the current health status of a population and an ideal situation where everyone in that population would reach old age in full health. For each disease, DALYs are calculated on a population scale as the sum of years lost due to premature mortality (YLL) and the healthy years lost due to disability.

Capability The knowledge, skills and experience of the staff of an institution and the procedural framework that allows the staff to operate as efficiently as possible.

Capacity The resources available to an institution in terms of staff, equipment, infrastructure and finance.

Jurisdiction Institutional power to regulate or control a project or particular aspects of a project.

Communicable diseases Diseases that are transmitted from a person or animal to another via a range of pathways, that include aerosols and droplets, contaminated water, food or materials, insects or intermediate hosts (as opposed to noncommunicable diseases, which do not spread from one individual to another).

Cost–effectiveness The analysis of cost–effectiveness is essentially a method of economic evaluation to compare different ways of achieving the same goal, by measuring costs in monetary terms and effects in physical units (such as reduction in incidence, or loss of disability-adjusted life years averted).

Cost–benefit The analysis of cost–benefit is another method of economic evaluation, which expresses both costs and benefits in monetary terms and therefore enables one to assess whether a particular objective is worth achieving.

Cross-cutting issues Issues of concern to more than one sector.

Environmental management for vector control The planning, organization, carrying out and monitoring of activities for the modification and/or manipulation of environmental factors or their interaction with humans with a view to preventing or minimizing vector propagation and reducing human–vector–pathogen contact.

Epidemiology The study of the geography, frequency, and environmental behavioural and social causes of disease transmission.

Feasibility A measure to prove that technical options are sustainable and the best in a given situation.

Health "Health is a state of complete physical, mental and social well-being and not merely the absence of disease or infirmity." (WHO Constitution, 1948).

Health hazard A health hazard is an agent that may cause harm (i.e. *Plasmodium* parasites which cause malaria).

Health risk A health risk is a measure of likelihood that an identified hazard causes harm to a particular group of people at a particular time and place (i.e. the risk that an imported case of malaria causes harm through natural transmission is nil in the absence of the *Anopheles* vector; increased humidity in an irrigation scheme can prolong the lifespan of *Anopheles* mosquitoes and increase the risk of malaria).

Health status The state of health of a person or population assessed with reference to morbidity, impairments, anthropological measurements, mortality, and indicators of functional status and quality of life.

Impact assessment The process of identifying the future consequences of a current or proposed action.

Environmental impact assessment The identification of future consequences of development on environmental parameters.

Health impact assessment A combination of procedures, methods, and tools by which a policy, programme or project may be judged as to its potential effects on the health of a population, and the distribution of those effects within the population.

Health management plan Intersectoral action plan for the implementation of agreed recommendations of an Environmental Health Impact Assessment, with intervention, health monitoring and compliance monitoring components, and usually supported by a Memorandum of Understanding (MoU) between the partners.

Incidence The number of cases of specific diseases diagnosed or reported during a defined period of time, divided by the number of persons making up the population in which they occurred.

Prevalence The number of people suffering from a specific disease at a particular moment in time in a defined population.

Internal rate of return The discount rate that makes the net present value of the stream of net benefits equal zero. The higher the internal rate of return (IRR), the more worthwhile the project.

Mitigation Implementation of measures that reduce harm.

Safeguards Measures that prevent harm.

Policy A course of action adopted by an authority for the achievement of an objective, guided by well-defined criteria for decision-making.

Strategy The allocation and deployment of resources and the establishment of institutional arrangements in pursuit of a policy.

Programme A definite plan of intended procedure with measurable targets within a realistic time frame.

Project Within a development programme, projects are the "units" of activities leading to a specific goal.

Project cycle A schematic representation of the sequence of actions required to initiate a project and complete it to its operational phase, whereby the output of each distinct phase is the input of the next phase.

Scavengers Marginalized people who perform in the informal sector of waste management and recycling.

Scoping A process of defining which communities, hazards, geographical areas and project phases should be included in an impact assessment.

Screening A process of sorting project proposals as part of an initial environmental examination to ascertain the need for health impact assessment.

Zoonosis An infectious disease transmissible under natural conditions from animals to humans.